Real Health, Real Life

JILLIAN LAMBERT, MS

FITNESS/NUTRITION/WELLNESS EXPERT

Real Health, Real Life
by Jillian Lambert, MS
Fitness/Nutrition/Wellness Expert
http://realhealthreallife.net/

Copyright 2012 by Jillian Lambert, MS
All rights reserved.
ISBN: 1466392312
ISBN 13: 9781466392311
Library of Congress Control Number: 2011917997
CreateSpace, North Charleston, SC

WHAT PEOPLE ARE
SAYING ABOUT JILLIAN

"Jillian Lambert has been my personal fitness trainer for over four years. Despite my busy career schedule, she has enabled me to maintain a healthy, balanced lifestyle. She gives me the motivation to exercise consistently and educated me on proper diet and nutrition. She is dependable, hardworking, and committed to helping me reach my fitness goals—not just for the short term, but for years to come." ~ Courtney Dudley, MD

"Jillian Lambert is our Feng Shui guru. She has an amazing aura of positive energy and her knowledge of Feng Shui runs deep. When she visited our home, my husband and I were very impressed with her thorough exploration of the house, inside and out, and her keen but gentle criticisms of our Feng Shui mistakes. Jillian gave us verbal and written suggestions with lots of specifics to help us achieve better Chi. It worked! We noticed a smoother flow in our home which led to a calmer existence and better productivity. It's difficult to describe, but definitely a welcomed change. Jillian's expertise is invaluable and I would recommend her services to anyone looking for all good things in life." ~ Karen Nugent, RN

WHAT PEOPLE ARE
SAYING ABOUT REAL HEALTH,
REAL LIFE

"What a treat it was reading Jillian Lambert's book *Real Health, Real Life*. It is obvious she has spent many years in this field trying different healthy ways of living and the reader is blessed to be able to learn from her experiences. I find many books on wellness difficult to read because they are either too verbose or I cannot relate to the stratospheric standards they encourage. Jillian's book is engaging, full of useful information, and like she says—for *real* people living typical (if there is such thing!) lives. It is refreshing to read a book on fitness with chapters about how to get back on the wagon once you have fallen off! Bravo!

I especially liked the chapters relating to emotional and spiritual wellness. Once again, Jillian shares her own experiences and gives many different options relating to healing those areas of our lives. I found those chapters to be delightful and extremely helpful.

Jillian has created a text that truly is holistic in every way—physically, mentally, emotionally, and spiritually. This book is applicable to anyone seeking healing or help in developing healthy practices in their lives. I commend her on this first effort and hope there are other books in her future written in this engaging, practical way!" ~ Lisa Powell-Watts, MEd, licensed professional counselor

"Praise to Jillian Lambert for finally writing a book I can understand and enjoy reading. I never had to go on a diet until I reached the age of forty. I then quit smoking and began menopause, which all resulted in me gaining twenty-five pounds. I didn't know what to do to get my life back together. I started reading Jillian's book *Real Health Real Life* and it all started making sense to me. She is a walking dictionary on your body's physical and emotional health and her Real Health Tips are easy to understand that you'll want to use them every day.

In her book, she is very compassionate and understands that we are all human and we will make mistakes along the way. Most health books are very clinical, but Jillian bares all to her readers which is why it is such a credible read. She is a talented writer and a dedicated wellness expert." ~Renee N., Southlake, TX

"If a person can't get motivated after reading this book, they may never do so. Jillian shares her vast experience in the fitness and nutrition world, as well as her life-long growth, emotionally, spiritually, and soulfully. After reading this, a person has to be able to identify with and be able to adopt a few of the many "exercises" she explains in her book. There are not many people who have experienced this many areas of self-improvement/growth…or someone who can open their soul and share this wealth of knowledge so that others may benefit. Simply amazing." ~ T.J. Jurica, health and fitness enthusiast

IN LOVING MEMORY OF MY MOTHER,
SHARON MOSBARGER,
WHO WAS A
BEAUTIFUL SOUL AND INSPIRATION.

This book would not be, if not for the love, warmth, and guidance of my mother, who helped me develop a passion for nutrition, fitness, and wellness. She was the one who answered all of my nutrition questions growing up.

She was the one who continued to exercise as long as she physically could.

She was the one who never gave up on her constant battle of weight loss…the one who successfully lost 130 pounds.

She was the one who never stopped reading books, watching Oprah, and learning about health and wellness.

She was the one who inspired me to not live life in fear.

She was the one who inspired me to express my feelings…speak my truth…and honor my soul.

My mother—the one who inspired me to live, love and learn.

ACKNOWLEDGMENTS

First and foremost, I would like to thank God, Jesus, Archangel Michael, the seraphim, my angels and guides for helping me to create this book. I have been inspired and guided by them all and am filled with great gratitude.

I graciously thank my mother for inspiring me regarding nutrition, fitness, and education…for being a beautiful listener and my emotional support over the years…for helping to instill within me a desire to read, learn, live, and grow… And my father, for his nonstop strength and for doing everything he could to care for my mother until the very end. I would also like to thank my intelligent, beautiful, and loving daughter, Brooke, who has blessed me with the honor of motherhood…for the times of "excitement" that made me laugh until I cried and the many times she touched my heart.

I express gratitude to my friends, family, sister Jan, past boyfriends, and ex-husband for our relationships and learning life experiences.

My gratitude to all the practitioners that helped to heal and educate me about holistic healing.

I am very grateful to Bernie and Stacy at Millennium 3 Education for creating a safe place to heal and grow emotionally. I also thank all of the staff for their volunteer work that supported me and many others through many personal growth trainings.

I offer gratitude to my spiritual friends who were there for me through good and challenging times. To those who were there for me, whether it be recently or over the years.

Angel Tom; glorious Chip; personal growth and spirit friend Wendy N.; giving, nonjudgmental Kathryn; dear, sweet chakra healer and supporter Lisa; my guides Carol and Diane; Zippity-Doo-Da Danny; big-hearted Sandi; respectful friend TJ; purest-of-hearts Georgy; my spiritual friend and client Courtney; retreat partner and spirit friend Kay and Silver Spur Ranch staff; dear soul friend and editor Pam; 2-steppin' Forrest, Gilbert, Buffalo Len, Larry, Tall Tom, Phyllis, "Energetic" Vicki, uplifting soul sister Nancy, the staff at OST, and the good people of Bandera, high energy Carrie; sweet, supportive Adrian; "fearsome foursome" friends Kari, Tracy, and Renee; entertaining and larger-than-life Darlene and Karen who made me laugh; soul dancer Mari; dear, country friend Nancy; good energy Rommy; yoga Susan; long-time friend Tamara; soul coach/friend Kellie; supportive EFT Kay; healer friend Tamie; my God-loving cousin Tony and Aunt Connie; Rancher Tiggs; Cowboy Alan; my healing horse friend, Ike; and my unconditionally loving cats, angel kitty Cairo and Journey.

And last but not least, my two dear soul sisters Joi and Wendy P. for all of their emotional support, guidance, acceptance, and unconditional love.

INTRODUCTION

This book is called *Real Health, Real Life*. The book is about being *real*, in health and in life. Being real means being true, or being honest, with yourself and with others.

It is not about being perfect. This is not one of those "perfect" fitness, nutrition or wellness books. You know what I mean: the books and authors that make you feel like you are a failure if you don't follow their steps to perfection. The world tends to promote perfectionism as having the perfect body, eating the perfect foods, and never going off course but staying on track and living the perfect life at all times.

Well, our bodies do not always look perfect, and we do not all eat perfectly at all times. And we don't all have the perfect life at all times.

Real health is not about eating the perfect number of calories every day to maintain your perfect muscle definition and perfect body. It's not about exercising every day for 45.2 minutes to maintain that perfect body.

Real health involves getting off track and sometimes not exercising because you overslept and didn't have time in the morning before work, or you chose not to exercise due to the depression you've been in since your mother died. *Real health* is about sometimes eating junk food because life got off track. Maybe you lost your job, lost someone you loved, or got divorced.

Real health takes into consideration that you may not feel like getting up and moving your body. Some days, you may be lucky just to get your body from the bed to the shower or make yourself go to work.

Real health is about fitness, nutrition, and wellness, but it is also about life experiences, our feelings, and how we deal with them. The most important aspect of *real health* is not how perfectly we stay on track, but that we *get back on* track. That is what we need to place importance on, not judging ourselves for falling off track, but *congratulating* ourselves for getting back on track.

Besides, who do you respect more—a woman whose body is genetically blessed and does nothing to maintain her genetically perfect body? Or the woman who is *not* genetically blessed, but keeps exercising and eating healthy—even if she falls off track 102 times, but still pulls herself up and gets back on track?

Do you respect the man who has the perfect job, perfect car, and trophy wife, who is trying to make a statement to the world that he indeed is perfect, only to find that behind the scenes, he lied and cheated to get that perfect job, does not own his car, and because of his lies to himself and others, his trophy wife actually cannot stand him? Or do you respect the man who lives a life he loves because he's passionate about it, respects himself and others, and most of all, honors his soul?

I know who I respect more.

Now let me be clear. I am grateful for the genetically perfect people here on earth. They give us all an image to aspire to, to get in shape and to improve ourselves. I just hope we do it in a healthful way, and for the right reasons. Not for egoism, impressing others, or to get attention or love from others.

What it comes down to is acceptance: acceptance of our bodies, ourselves, and who we are. We are all unique individuals. Real life is about acknowledging that: accepting that we are all special in our own way. Developing our inner beauty is more important than developing our outer beauty.

Ha! Good luck with that in this society, right?

I know. I tried to be "Little Miss Perfect" for many years. The message regarding perfection was delivered when I was a young girl, it grew in adolescence, and finally came to a head in adulthood. First it was about getting braces, then contact lenses, and all the "right" clothes. Later in life, it was the "right" husband, big house, nice car, and finally, a breast augmentation. All of this because I wanted to be perfect. Growing up, I received the message from home and people in society that "if you are perfect, you will be loved."

So, I did whatever I could within my power to look perfect: my hair, makeup, body, clothes, and so on. The list goes on and on…and then you want to puke.

The funny thing is, back then I didn't think anything of it. I was just doing what I felt I was supposed to do to be accepted and to be loved. Now, looking back, I realize it is about *me* accepting myself and *me* loving myself, not trying to *get* acceptance and love *from others*.

Real health starts with YOU accepting you and loving you.

You loving yourself. Not through perfectionism, fake-ism, and the facade of how perfect we all want to be, but *realistic* health and the creation of a *realistic* life.

I am not talking about surgery. I tried that route. It changes the outside of you but does not enhance your inner beauty. After many years of physical, emotional, and spiritual detox, I can tell you it is a much better investment to enhance your inner beauty. The external beauty fades, but the inner beauty shines on. Yes, looking and feeling good physically feels great, but don't stop there. Life gets better when you take on beauty depth: your inner beauty. It is about loving your body, yourself, and your soul.

I write this to you through realness, honesty, and truth. I hope you take something from this book that in some way benefits you, your life, your overall wellness, and *realness*.

In health, healing, and realness,
Jillian Lambert ☺

CONTENTS

SECTION I:

REAL NUTRITION

REAL FOOD

This book is based on various wellness practices I have experienced and believe in. This book has been written to help you create *real health* for yourself. You are the one in charge of your life. You are the one in charge of your health. You CAN improve your health. Your overall health is in YOUR hands. You can use your body, mind, and spirit to reshape it, re-create it and rejuvenate it.

How? By eating *real food* and drinking *real juice.*

What is *real food*? I don't think we know anymore. We have been buying and eating food made by man for too many years. We have been consuming chemicals, additives, preservatives, hormones, and pesticides. We are eating poisons. We are killing ourselves. Cancer is everywhere because chemicals are everywhere: in our food, the air we breathe, the water we drink, and the products we use.

Real food is about getting back to basics. *Real food* is about plants and nature...not labs and factories. *Real food* is about healing our bodies...not poisoning them.

GETTING BACK TO BASICS

Whenever you question whether something is good for you, think "caveman"...think "earth"...think "plants"...think "nature." Ask yourself: "Did cavemen eat this?"

BOXES, CANS, AND BAGS

Here is another way to look at it. Before you put anything in your mouth, think. I mean really think. Did this come in a bag? Did this come in a box? Did this come in a can? If it came in a bag, think *body bag*. If it came in a box, think *coffin*. If it came in a can, think *trash can*. Anything that did not come in a bag, box or can is pretty much *real* food.

MICROWAVES

Are microwaves a healthy way to prepare food? There is reason to believe that microwaves could change the molecular structure of our food. Because of this, your body does not know what to do with the "changed" food. We do not know how the body reacts to microwaved food on a molecular level. Because of this, it is safer to avoid using your microwave. If you need to cook something, I recommend using an oven, stove top, or broiler. If you feel you must use a microwave, the less often you use it, the better.

PLANTS AND NATURE

Ask yourself: "Did this come from the earth?" *Real food* starts with fruits and vegetables, and fruits and vegetables start with dirt. Fruits and vegetables come from the earth: dirt.

ORGANIC

If the food did come from the ground, ask:

"Was it sprayed with chemicals?"

"Is it clean?"

Real fruits and vegetables are organic (pesticide-free), fresh, and whole. (Whole, being the fruit or vegetable is in its natural state, without being cooked or processed.) Go for the vegetables that are grown fresh locally, in your garden, or in the organic section of your supermarket. Organic fruits and vegetables are higher priced, but they are also higher in vitamins and minerals. So you are getting more for your money when you buy organic.

RAW VS. COOKED

Raw foods are not cooked. A food is "cooked" when it is heated at the temperature of 118 °F or higher. Enzyme damage *starts* at 104 °F, and *destroyed* at 118 degrees Fahrenheit, according to David Wolfe, author of *The Sunfood Diet Success System.* If you want to preserve the enzymes in your food, do not cook it over 118 degrees Fahrenheit. Have you ever noticed how much better you feel after eating a lot of salads, fresh fruit, and raw vegetables? That's because those raw fruits and vegetables have "live" enzymes, according to Dr. Edward Howell, author of *Enzyme Nutrition.*

RAW FOODISM

A raw foodist is someone who eats a high raw diet—or even 100 percent—raw food diet. A raw food diet usually consists of raw fruits, vegetables, nuts and seeds, no animal products, nothing cooked. The reason people do this is to feel good and experience excellent health. In the past, I have been a meat and potatoes person, a vegetarian, a vegan, and a raw foodist. I was a raw foodist for two years and felt absolutely incredible—the best I have ever felt physically. It felt like a natural high. So many positive changes occurred in my health. My skin looked great, my eyes were bright, I had no body odor, no "sleep" in the corners of my eyes in the mornings. I became extremely lean, and slept deeper and for fewer hours. I had a ton of energy, never got sick, and if injured from exercise, I healed ten times quicker than when I was a non-raw foodist.

When I was a raw foodist, even my eyesight improved!

So, why did I stop being 100 percent raw? I had been extremely disciplined in my eating, for years and years. At age forty, I decided that I missed eating salmon and incorporated it back into my diet. Salmon is my favorite kind of protein, and my body metabolizes it very well. Another reason I stopped being 100 percent raw is that it was a bit challenging to do in this country. I decided that I could eat a high raw diet and still enjoy foods I missed that were still good for my body.

ENZYMES

What are enzymes? They are protein chemicals that our bodies need in order to function. Dr. Edward Howell, author of *Enzyme Nutrition*, states that, "Enzymes are substances that make life possible. They are needed for every chemical reaction that takes place in the human body. No mineral, vitamin, or hormone can do any work without enzymes. Our bodies, all our organs, tissues, and cells are run by metabolic enzymes." They help us breathe, exercise, and digest. There are three kinds: metabolic, digestive, and food enzymes. Metabolic enzymes help in motor functions (i.e. blinking the eyes, turning the head, etc.) Digestive enzymes help break down and digest foods. There are also food enzymes in *raw* foods.

Anytime you cook fruits and vegetables over 118 °F, you destroy the "live" food enzymes. Yep, "dead" enzymes are what you've got. Dead enzymes create *dead food* and don't do much good for your body. "Live" enzymes are a different story. When you eat raw foods, you are actually putting "life" into your body. That's why you feel lighter, happier and healthier when you eat more salads, fresh fruits and raw vegetables. Want to feel sluggish? Cook'em.

David Wolfe, raw food expert, states that "Enzymes are vital to all life processes. Enzymes are catalysts for all reactions in the body. They embody the vital Sun energy in the body—they are transformers directed by hormones amongst a terrain of vitamins, minerals, carbohydrates, fats and tissue proteins."

Dr. Edward Howell, who wrote *Enzyme Nutrition*, had a theory regarding enzymes. He believed that we are all born with a certain amount of enzymes in our bodies. We use these enzymes up as we age. Once we are out of enzymes, we die. The more enzymes we can preserve, the longer we live, the better we look, and the healthier we feel.

Think of your body as a bank. Think of your enzymes as money. Every time you eat raw foods, you make a deposit into your bank. Every time you put cooked or processed food into your body, you make a withdrawal from your bank. It is considered a withdrawal because your body has to pull from its own storage of digestive enzymes to digest any cooked or processed foods. Raw foods, on the other hand, are considered a deposit, since they have "live" enzymes to help digest themselves. This "help" to the digestive system frees up energy. So, next time you put something in your mouth, ask yourself if you are making a deposit or a withdrawal.

If you are going to eat cooked food, consider taking enzyme capsules before eating your *dead food*. You can get enzyme capsules at any health food store. I like to use LifeZymes by Harvey Diamond or Pure Encapsulations Digestive Enzymes Ultra. *(Note: I do not benefit in any way financially from the recommendation of these products.)*

VITAMINS AND MINERALS

Vitamins and minerals are important to our bodies. Vitamins and minerals help the body's cells and organs function properly. The category of foods that contain the most minerals and second most vitamins are vegetables. The category of foods that contain the most vitamins and second most minerals are fruits.

There are two types of vitamins: fat-soluble and water-soluble. Fat-soluble vitamins, K,A,D, and E can be stored within the body for longer amounts than water-soluble. Water-soluble vitamins, B and C, need to be replenished on a regular basis. These vitamins become depleted due to stress, alcohol, smoking, and exercise, so the body needs to have a constant supply.

Calcium is a mineral that helps in many body functions. Bone building and muscle contraction are just two. Calcium comes from sources such as dark leafy greens (spinach, romaine lettuce, celery, chard, broccoli), tomatoes, figs, grapefruit, honeydew melons, peaches, pineapples, strawberries, and dairy.

Dairy products are the first foods that most people think of when considering calcium. Dairy does contain a high amount of calcium, but is also acidic to the body. Not only is dairy acidic, but can cause many other problems in the body (lactose intolerance, and so on).

Another source of calcium is soy milk. It too, is acidic, but is a plant-based food. It is high in calcium, low in fat, low in calories, low in carbs, and high in protein. Some people feel that soy milk has other issues (estrogen and thyroid issues, for instance) but it depends on the person and how their body processes it. Personally, I prefer soy milk and use it as my main source of calcium.

Rice milk and almond milk are less acidic and are healthy alternatives to dairy. Their protein content is not as high as that of soy milk, but diet needs differ. What do you need? More protein? Fewer carbs? Fewer calories? Less fat? More calcium?

ACID VS ALKALINE

The body needs to keep everything in balance to experience good health (this is called homeostasis). When the body consumes too many acidic foods and not enough alkaline foods, the body is out of balance. This imbalance weakens the body's ability to ward off infectious microorganisms. Acidic foods must be balanced with alkaline foods for *real health*.

You can use pH paper to test your alkaline level. Tear off a two to three inch strip of pH paper and place it under the stream of your urine during the first urination of the day. After making contact with your urine, the pH paper will turn color. Match the color of the paper to the graph on the pH paper container. This will tell you if you are alkaline or acidic. (For best health, your pH level should be in the range of 7.35-7.45). This is the level that helps the body fight off disease. When the body is out of balance, the immune system is compromised. This weakens the body's ability to fight off colds, flu, viruses and disease.

If too many acidic foods are consumed by the body, calcium is leached from the bones. Acidic foods include dairy, meats and many processed foods and beverages. Alkaline foods help neutralize the acid of acidic foods. Most raw fruits and vegetables and/or fresh juices are alkaline foods. If you have a high raw food diet (fifty percent or higher of raw fruits, vegetables and/or fresh juices), your pH reading is most likely going to be within a healthy alkaline range. For more information on the effects of acid and alkaline foods see *The Acid Alkaline Food Guide*, by Dr. Susan E. Brown and Larry Trivieri, Jr.

SUPPLEMENTS

Supplements can add what may be missing from your diet. Supplements, like anything else, can be overdone or underdone. The supplements I feel are important are B complex, calcium, mixed greens supplement, and digestive enzymes to make digestion easier when eating cooked foods.

A multivitamin can also be very beneficial to make sure you are getting all the vitamins and minerals your body needs. Everyone has a different body with different deficiencies, so make sure you supplement your body as needed.

I stick to raw fruits and vegetables as much as possible. When I do eat cooked food, I always take a digestive enzyme supplement before my cooked meal. Depending on the brand, enzyme supplements are taken before, during, or after the meal. However, when I eat a 100 percent raw food meal, I skip the enzyme supplement. Supplementing with digestive enzyme supplements makes a huge difference in digestion and how you feel after eating a cooked meal. Enzymes help make digestion less taxing on the body.

Another way to help with the body's digestion is to eat raw foods or a salad with every cooked meal. The live enzymes within the raw vegetables help digest the cooked food. Enzymes also help the body eliminate anything the body does not need. Elimination is a way of cleansing the body.

REAL JUICE

When juicing, make sure you drink the juice soon after juicing the fruit or vegetables to receive all of the medicinal properties. If you wait too long before drinking the fresh juice, oxidation sets in and can rob you of important vitamins, minerals, and enzymes. Oxidation occurs when free radicals attack the juice (or food) and kill the live enzymes in your fresh juice, fruits and vegetables. Cooler temperatures (refrigeration) can slow the oxidation process and help the medicinal properties last longer, but it's always best to drink immediately after juicing.

Juices on the shelf in the grocery store are dead. There are no live enzymes in store-bought juice, unless it is labeled. Juices in the store have been pasteurized; they have been heated (or cooked) to a temperature over 118 °F, which disqualifies it from the definition of raw food.

In other words, when you buy juice from the store, you are drinking dead juice. You may get some vitamins out of the dead juice, but usually it's because vitamins have been added back in. Live enzymes are what give you "life." Dead juice has no enzymes and gives you empty calories, unless fortified.

The reason food companies pasteurize juice is to kill any bacteria that may be in the fresh juice. Yes, there is a slight chance of bacterial contamination, but it is unlikely. Bacteria can be on anything, anytime, anywhere. The food companies pasteurize the juice for fear of someone getting sick. The way I look at it is if you want to live your life in fear, go for it. The chances of getting sick are similar from touching a doorknob or someone sneezing on you.

What it comes down to is your immune system. If you have a healthy immune system, you can fight off germs, bacteria, and other pathogens. I drink pasteurized juice just as a beverage on occasion, but I do not drink dead juice for health benefits.

Freezing can also rob fruits and vegetables of live enzymes. Freezing fresh foods or juice can kill 30 percent of the live enzymes. This is why it is best to eat fresh whole fruits, vegetables and juices.

JUICING FOR HEALTH

Juicing is great for cleansing your body and for when you are sick. Juicing is a great way to get more vitamins and minerals into your body. If you are sick or coming down with something, juicing is a good way to stop the illness before it becomes full-blown and it helps to relieve the body from the taxing work of digestion.

Digestion takes a large amount of energy. That is why a lot of people do not have an appetite when sick. It is their body's way of taking the energy from digestion and putting it toward healing. Juicing helps pump vitamins and minerals into the body, yet frees up energy for the healing process. The body becomes more efficient and recovery time is much quicker.

I have used juicing to stave off a cold, flu, and other illnesses. Usually, juicing stops it in its tracks. Whenever I feel a sore throat coming on, I juice several grapefruit. The fresh juice makes my throat feel better and usually helps heal it completely.

When someone has a high temperature, appetite is usually low. High body temperature helps kill bacteria. The body has its ways of healing itself; we tend to get in the way of that sometimes. I am not telling you to avoid medical help. Seek medical advice from your holistic or healthcare professional, but also listen to your body. If you are sick and do not feel like eating, listen to your body. It knows best. If you are feeling weak and hungry, by all means eat. Many times when someone is sick, it is due to the body being in need of a cleanse.

REAL INTERNAL
HEALTH/DETOX

Today's American diet is full of sugar, nutrient-depleted flour, fatty meats, processed foods, and fried foods. There are many preservatives and chemicals that decrease your body's ability to cleanse itself. These preservatives and chemicals also slow the digestion process. When digestion slows down, it creates a clogging of your system. According to the internal health clinic I worked with, the colon becomes clogged and breeds bacteria, parasites, and worms that are damaging. This damage sets up an environment for disease. One way to ensure internal health is to cleanse (detox) your system.

REAL CLEANSING/ ELIMINATION

CLEANSING/DETOX

Everybody is so concerned about how they look on the outside. We go to great lengths to bathe, wash our hair, curl it, put on makeup, brush our teeth, and spend tons of money on various creams, lotions, and moisturizers to make sure that we look presentable.

The smell of our bodies is also a concern with us. We go to great lengths to make sure our bodies smell clean even though they may not be clean on the inside. We spend so much money on antiperspirants, deodorants, toothpaste, mouthwash and mints, feminine sprays, colognes, and perfumes just to make sure we smell good.

Why don't we take the same amount of time, money, and energy to clean the inside of our bodies? Because we don't know what it looks like or smells like on the inside of our bodies. If we did, we would definitely think twice about what we put into our bodies.

I find it funny that we are so concerned about changing the oil in our cars every three to seven thousand miles to make sure our car runs well, but we don't think about how to make our bodies run well. We would never consider putting ten or fifteen gallons of sugar in the gas tanks of our cars, yet we put at least that much sugar into our bodies every year. I'm not saying that I haven't eaten sugar before, but I will tell you, it's something to think about.

Here are three reasons to cleanse your body: parasites, Candida, and worms. Most people have at least one of these within their body and/or colon. It's pretty disgusting to think about, but I worked in an internal health clinic and I am telling you it's true. We may not want to believe it or accept it, but there are a lot of uncomfortable issues going on inside our bodies; I've seen them. I'm not sure if it's a good thing, not to be able to see what goes on inside our bodies. We would take much better care of our bodies if we were able to see inside them.

After years of putting chemicals, hormones, preservatives, additives, and pesticides into your body, it is a good idea to cleanse your body. Once your body is cleansed, it can then take in *real food* and start the healing/rebuilding process. If your body is toxic from eating junk over the years, it is probably not absorbing much of the nutrients from the *real food* you are eating! According to the internal health clinic I worked with, a coating of chemicals, hormones, preservatives, additives and pesticides develops along the lining of the colon. This coating appears to block or decrease the absorption of valuable nutrients. After you cleanse the body and feed it *real food*, the *real food* is then absorbed at a much higher rate.

There are all sorts of ways to cleanse your body internally. There are juice fasts, water fasts, and raw fruit and vegetable fasts. There are liver cleanses, gallbladder cleanses, colonics...the list goes on. Some cleanses are more potent and detox the body more quickly. Other detox formulas work at a slower rate. The slower the cleanse, the milder the detox symptoms. Of course, the stronger the cleanse, the stronger the detox symptoms.

Detox symptoms affect some people, but not others. It all depends on you and how toxic your body is. Detox symptoms can include any of the following:

* fatigue
* headache
* light-headedness
* nausea
* irritability
* diarrhea

Your body may experience any (or none) of these symptoms. Usually symptoms last anywhere from one to three days. Just know that if your body experiences them, it is usually a good thing. Your body is releasing all of the toxins from your body so it can replace them with healthy nutrients. Most times a slow, mild cleanse is less shocking to the body, giving it a chance to adjust without disrupting your activities.

After your body is cleansed, the healing and rebuilding process can begin. Your body is constantly producing new cells. According to the internal health clinic I worked at, if the body has unhealthy cells to work with, it can only produce more unhealthy cells. If your body has healthy cells to work with, then it can produce more healthy cells. Eating *real food* will help your body create healthy cells. The healthy cells have a better chance at reproducing if the old, unhealthy cells are cleaned out first. So cleanse your body and eat *real food*.

CLEANSE/DETOX MENU

Eating a clean diet of *real foods* before your cleanse is a way of preparing your body for detoxification. A pre-cleanse diet three to seven days prior can help decrease detox symptoms.

It is just as important to add regular foods back into your diet s-l-o-w-l-y *after* detoxification! Ease your body back into solid foods with *real foods*. For example, begin your post-cleanse eating with fruits for one or two days, then add vegetables only for a day or two. About five to seven days after the end of your cleanse, you can add grains to your diet (such as brown rice or spelt pasta) for a day or two, then move into meats, beginning with fish, then turkey and/or chicken, and finally beef. Adding regular foods back into your diet as listed here helps the body adjust to digestion mode again. If you do a cleanse and then jump right into eating something difficult to digest like meats—especially beef—it is a shock to your system and you may experience physical discomfort such as fatigue, headache, nausea, or light-headedness.

Sample menu for 1–2 weeks prior to cleanse (reproduced as a handout in Appendix)

BREAKFAST
Lemon water upon rising
Fresh, whole, raw fruit and/or fresh juice (preferably organic fruit)
Any fresh fruit (not dried fruit), throughout morning

LUNCH
Organic Vegetarian Sandwich
    2 slices Ezekiel Organic Sprouted Grain Bread
    1/2 ripe avocado (may substitute flaxseed oil or
        coconut oil)
    organic tomato slices
    organic baby carrots cut in half (length-wise)

organic cucumber slices (skin cut off unless organic)

organic yellow bell pepper slices (1/4–1/3 section of
bell pepper)

2–3 organic romaine lettuce leaves

(Or other variety of fresh, raw vegetables)

Lightly toast Ezekiel bread. Spread avocado or oil onto toast and top with vegetables.

-OR-

PROTEIN LUNCH

Organic Turkey Wraps (may substitute with lean ground beef, chicken or tuna)

4–6 fresh, organic romaine lettuce leaves

3–5 oz. free-range, hormone-free lean cooked turkey

organic vegetable mix: 2–3 preferably raw green
vegetables (or lightly steamed)

Wash lettuce leaves. Use each leaf like a taco shell, filling with turkey and raw veggies.

DINNER

Free-Range Grilled Chicken Salad (may substitute any lean meat such as lean ground beef, turkey, or salmon)

1 free-range chicken breast

Mrs. Dash or healthy seasoning

Organic spring salad mix

Raw or lightly steamed green veggies (broccoli,
green beans, etc.)

Sprinkle seasoning on chicken. Bake or grill until cooked thoroughly. Slice or chop chicken breast and arrange over spring salad mix.

For more recipes, see Real Recipes *in the Appendix.*

CLEANSING WITH JUICE

Juicing is a great way to cleanse your body. Doing a juice cleanse gives your body a break from the heavy task of digestion and feeds your body many vitamins and minerals. I did a nine-day juice cleanse and felt incredible for most of it. There were times when I felt tired and had a slight headache, but that was within the first two to three days. The fatigue and headache were detox symptoms. I did not experience the light-headedness, irritability, and nausea detox symptoms. The fatigue and headache was my body's way of eliminating toxins that had built up over a period of time. I have done many different cleanses. Each cleanse was a different experience.

How toxic your body is determines how you feel on a cleanse. If you have been eating a healthy, clean diet, then you can expect fewer symptoms during the cleanse. On the other hand, if you have been feeding your body with junk for a long period of time, then you may experience more severe detox symptoms.

Cleaning out your body can be as simple as taking some cleansing capsules from a health food store. I personally don't feel that this is as effective as other cleanses, but it is a nice place to start if you have never done an internal cleanse. Juicing is, I believe, more effective and sure to fill your body with "live" enzymes.

Another option is to buy fresh juice from a health food store. The cleanse I like to do is a citrus cleanse consisting of grapefruit, oranges, and lemons.

Select a two-day period when you have a light schedule to do a cleanse. On these days, drink eight ounces every hour (in place of food) from morning until evening. Light exercise is okay, just don't overdo it. Please listen to your body. Consult a health care professional before doing any type of cleanse. Be prepared for possible detox symptoms.

2-DAY DETOX CLEANSE
(reproduced as a handout in Appendix)

> 6 large grapefruit
>
> 8 large oranges or tangerines
>
> 4 lemons
>
> 1/2–1 gallon of purified water
>
> 1 juicer or juice extractor (brands include Juiceman Juicer, Champion, and others)

Cut away the surface of the peels of the grapefruit, oranges, and lemons, leaving the white pith on the fruit. (It contains bio-flavonoids: plant chemicals that help with absorption of vitamin C in citrus fruit). Cut fruit in quarters and put through juicer (with a large enough container under it to hold the juice). Mix juice with 1/2 gallon of purified water. (If you want the juice to last longer, mix with 1 whole gallon of purified water.) Keep refrigerated.

OTHER AREAS TO DETOX:

Note that as you cleanse your body, you may find a desire to detox/cleanse your home, emotions and/or your relationships. (See Relationships and Emotional Health section. For home detox, see Feng Shui section.)

THE BODY'S SEWER SYSTEM

How many times a day do you go to the bathroom? If you eat two to three times a day but only go to the bathroom once, food gets backed up. In my experience working at an internal health clinic, your colon can accumulate up to six to nine rotting meals in your system. If you are not eliminating two to three times a day, the waste rots and creates toxins.

Tip: When going to the bathroom, place your feet up on something like a foot stool or wastebasket.   Raising your knees above your hips while eliminating helps create more thorough elimination.

Your colon is the sewer system of your body. Your digestive tract is twelve times the length of your body! What happens when this long digestive tract gets backed up? It is like a toilet that is backed up. The waste has nowhere to go, so it overflows. It's the same in your colon, except instead of overflowing onto the floor, it gets pumped back into your bloodstream. The toxins are reabsorbed into your body; they can compromise your immune system and make you more vulnerable to disease. While working at an internal health clinic, I learned that nearly 90 percent of all degenerative diseases start in the colon.

The toxins that are pumped back into your body make you feel tired, achy, nauseous, and irritable. A toxic colon becomes a breeding ground for parasites, yeast infections, tumors, worms, and disease. If not released, these issues can turn into bigger problems such as fissures, hemorrhoids, polyps, and possibly cancer. Toxins create disease, or autointoxication. Autointoxication is self-intoxication: poisoning the self with toxins.

Colonics don't sound so extreme now, do they? One of the most beneficial cleanses I have ever done for my body was a cleanse with nutritional shakes, herbs, supplements and colonics. I did a ten-day fast and felt like a million bucks! Even though I have eaten very healthy for the majority of my life, I was surprised at how much my body needed the cleanse. I found that I needed only five to six hours of sleep, had more energy, and felt relief of the aches in my knees. I even lost a few pounds!

The pounds I lost, I believe, were toxins that built up over the years. Those toxins were slowing me down and decreasing my energy. During and after the cleanse, my energy increased. Please note that I did experience detox symptoms such as nausea, light-headedness, and fatigue. There were also bouts of unbelievable energy! You don't have to do a ten-day cleanse. Start off with a one-day cleanse. Within one to three months you may want to work your way up to a three-, five-, or seven-day cleanse if you like. Remember that everyone's body is different and may respond to different cleanses differently.

Colonics are a small price to pay to detoxify your precious body. You only get one body, so love it by taking care of it and cleaning it.

COLONICS: GET IT IN, GET IT OUT

If you are really serious about cleansing your body, try a total body cleanse through colonics. Colonics include an internal cleansing of your colon or intestines. This may sound extreme, but this is where you get the *real cleaning* done in your body. Your colon is like a sewer system of the body. If foods are not chewed or digested properly, or are improperly combined, they remain stagnant in your intestines.

The goal of eating food is to get it in, process it, absorb the nutrients, and get it out. The sooner you get it out, the better. According to the book *Fit for Life*, food sits in that warm, moist environment, it putrefies, rots, and becomes extremely toxic. The longer undigested, or improperly digested food or toxins sit in the intestines, the more toxic your body becomes. This is why it is important to chew your food well and combine it with other compatible foods for proper digestion. This will improve nutrient absorption and proper elimination.

Note: Try to chew each bite of food fifty times to improve digestion and nutrient absorption.

The amount of time it takes to digest certain foods varies. Most fruits spend approximately thirty minutes in the stomach. Cantaloupe spends about fifteen to twenty minutes, while bananas can take up to forty-five minutes to an hour when eating fruit on an empty stomach.

Now, vegetables can take up to an hour and a half in the stomach. That is a shorter amount of time than for meat, which can take up to four hours—that is, if it is properly combined with vegetables. If you eat an improperly combined meal such as meat and starchy foods (potatoes, bread, rice, or pasta), it can take up to eight hours in the stomach! Most people are eating the next meal before the last meal has been digested!

Note: Make sure to take a probiotic supplement when doing colonics to replace any beneficial bacteria that may have been lost.

HOLISTIC HEALTH MACHINES
RIFE MACHINE

Another way to detox your body is with a Rife machine. You'll probably notice that I refer to my Rife machine throughout this book. This machine has been discussed in Kevin Trudeau's newsletter, The Lark Letter: Women's Guide to Optimal Health and the Well Being Journal. The machine generates five hundred fifty different frequencies to help you improve your health. I use my Rife machine two to three times a week just to detox. I could be detoxing pesticides, smog from my lungs, or any other toxins that may have entered my body. This machine sends a gentle electric frequency through the body to kill harmful micro-organisms. It does not harm the beneficial micro-organisms. The detoxification session takes approximately thirty-three minutes. I do a session when I have the time or when I am feeling sluggish. Drinking water after a session helps to flush out any die-off of micro-organisms or toxins.

The man who designed the machine, Dr. Royal Raymond Rife, went to great lengths to make this machine. According to the article "Dr. Royal Rife's Discovery Cures Cancers" in the *Well Being Journal*, Rife used his machine to help cure people with cancer and a long list of other ailments. Royal has since passed away, but his machine lives on. Look it up. Every household should have one. As I tell all my friends and family, if there were a fire and I could grab three items from my home, my Rife machine would definitely be one of them. I could go on and on about this incredible machine, but that would take a whole other book to write!

Note: Do not attempt to use a Rife machine or frequency generator if you are epileptic, pregnant or have a pacemaker/heart issues.

IONIC FOOT BATH

An ionic foot bath is a small device that is submerged into a tub of water and pulls toxins from the pores in your feet as you soak them. While working at an internal health clinic, I learned that this machine detoxifies your kidneys, bladder, urinary tract, female/prostrate area, gallbladder, joints, liver and lymphatic system. Your feet release many toxins ranging from Candida, alcohol, tobacco, dead blood cells, and various metals. As your feet soak in the tub of water you will see the water change color. The color of the water tells you what toxins your body is excreting.

When the color turns yellow-green, you are detoxifying from the kidneys, bladder, urinary tract, and female or prostate area. Orange water means you are detoxifying from your joints. Brown water means you are detoxifying your liver, tobacco and/or cellular debris. If you produce black water, you are also detoxifying from the liver. Dark green water means you are detoxifying from your gallbladder and lymphatic system (most likely yeast). Black flecks on top of the water indicate that heavy metals are being released. Red flecks at the top of the water reflect dead blood cell material.

If you decide to do an ionic foot bath with a friend (using separate machines and tubs), you may notice that your friend's water is a different color from yours. Don't be surprised if you come up orange and your friend comes up black! Everyone's body is different when detoxing.

It's actually fun to do this the first time, because it feels like magic. During the thirty-minute session, you can sit and watch the water turn colors. I thought the attendant put food coloring in my foot bath the first time I did it. It was amazing to see my feet produce colored water.

After a foot bath, you may feel a bit tired, or it may energize you. The first time I felt tired, but I felt great the next day. I have felt energized almost every time by the foot bath since then. Just remember that everyone is different, and be patient with yourself.

When I worked at the internal cleansing clinic, the machine's instructions recommended that foot baths should be done no more than once every two days. For full cleanses, they recommended doing a foot bath every other day for a month.

Once I did two foot baths back to back. I felt fine after the first one, but nauseated after the second. Thank God it was bedtime. I went straight to bed. Do not do what I did. I did this at a time when I had gotten off track with my *real healthy* eating and thought that if one foot bath was good, then two would be better. Not so—not in the same night, back to back. It was too much detoxing for my system to handle at the time.

Note: *Whenever you detox your body, you may experience some of the detox symptoms: nausea, light-headedness, headache, irritability, diarrhea, fatigue, and so on. Symptoms can vary depending on the type and extent of detox you are doing and how toxic your body is to begin with.*

Be aware that there are many types of ionic foot baths on the market and some are better models than others. Be sure to read the instructions, as they may differ from model to model. Some foot baths require sea salt to be added to the water while others require iodized salt. Some models have one foot bath unit; others have a dual unit where two people can take a foot bath at the same time. Each model may use different attachments, types of salt or wrist band to wear while using it. It all depends on what your needs are.

I have had a Q Live dual foot bath machine for several months now and it seems to work very well so far. My other model is called Bio-Cleanse Technology. I have had it for years. Check them out on the web and see what suits your needs. (See Ionic Foot Bath Chart in Appendix)

REAL ENERGY

Why settle for fake energy when you can have *real energy*? Don't rely on coffee, sodas, or other drinks with caffeine. Those drinks may give you a temporary boost, but eventually exhaust your body even more. They trick you and your body into believing that you have energy—and you do, for a short amount of time. You are much better off creating real sustained energy through *real foods*, *real juices*, and proper digestion.

You make less work for your body and have more energy when you eat raw or "live" foods. You free up energy that would have been used for digestion and it can now be used for other things—like thinking, exercising, playing with your kids, and so on. Notice that your exercise sessions are more energetic after eating some fresh fruit for breakfast versus how you feel after cooked eggs and bacon.

REAL LEAN

People are more weight-conscious today than ever before. This has caused many to lose sight of their *real beauty* in search of their ideal weight and a "perfect" body image. However, weight *is* important for *real health* and *real energy*.

ADDING LEANNESS

This section is called "Adding Leanness" for two reasons. First, this term is more positive than *weight loss*. Second, it's about adding or bringing something *to* your body and your life, not taking anything away. In other words, this way of eating is about bringing healthy foods and activities into your life. The focus is about adding in, not removal or deprivation.

If you have a goal to be healthy or lean, focus on the healthy foods you are adding to your way of eating. Focus on adding exercise. Focus on drinking more water. Drink ten to twelve ounces fifteen minutes before a meal and see how full you feel. Focus on adding soul activities. Focus on bringing more nature into your life. Focus on new projects and hobbies that support a healthy lifestyle. When you are focusing on all of the healthy things you are bringing in to your life, the not-so-healthy foods, activities and behaviors will eventually be squeezed out. You won't miss them as much and may not even notice they've disappeared!

DIETS

Whoa! Diet is a sore subject among most people! Yuck! Who likes to diet? Yes, it can be a bit exciting to start a new diet just because it is new and different. It can also be dangerous and restricting. I've tried all sorts of ways of eating. I've tried high-carb, low-carb, high-protein, low-protein, high-fat, low-fat, vegetarianism, pesco-vegetarianism (veggies and fish), ovo-vegetarianism (veggies and eggs), veganism (no animal products), and raw-foodism (no cooked food). Let me tell you, it's been exhausting and frustrating, yet interesting and educational. It's interesting to see how the body responds to different foods.

When trying out a new way of eating, you may want to ask yourself these five questions:

DOES IT MAKE SENSE?

If it is a Twinkie Diet...common sense should tell you that it's probably not a healthy way to eat.

DOES IT WORK?

If it works for other people, maybe there is something to it. But, that doesn't necessarily mean that it will work for you and your body.

IS IT SAFE?

If people are having unhealthy responses, it's probably not a good choice.

HOW DOES IT MAKE ME FEEL?

If you feel healthy and energized, then maybe it's for you. If you feel tired, sluggish, or weak, maybe it's not for you. Of course, those side effects may only be detox symptoms. If symptoms persist after three or four days, the diet may not be a good choice for you. *Please listen to your body.*

CAN I EAT THIS WAY LONG-TERM?

If you feel comfortable and healthy doing it long-term, then great. If not, then maybe you need to re-think it.

Whatever you decide to experiment with, please, please, please *listen to your body.*

You only get one body. Love it, listen to it, and respect it.

REAL WAYS OF EATING

WAYS OF EATING FOR REAL WEIGHT LOSS

There are all kinds of ways to eat. There are all kinds of ways to lose weight. There are all kinds of ways to eat healthy. Your job is to *find out what works for YOUR body.* Every body is different. Every body has different needs. What one body may respond to beautifully, another may reject. Get to know your body and feed it the way it needs to be fed. Here are some eating styles to try.

1. FRUIT UNTIL NOON

This way of eating is my favorite. I have been practicing it for twenty-one years, because it has worked wonderfully for me. I choose to eat this way for three reasons. First, it's very healthy and cleansing to my body. Second, it frees up energy, keeps me energized, and makes me feel great. Finally, it's easy and keeps my weight in check.

Why fruit until noon?

The book *Fit for Life, by* Harvey and Marilyn Diamond theorizes that our bodies go through three stages in a twenty-four-hour period. These are Appropriation, Assimilation, and Elimination.

The Appropriation (or Digestion) Stage usually takes place from 12:00 p.m. to 8:00 p.m. This is when your body digests food and beverages.

The second stage is the Assimilation Stage: 8:00 p.m. through 4:00 a.m. This is the time when your body absorbs all of the nutrients from the foods you have eaten. It will absorb whatever it is *able* to absorb, depending on the health of your body and digestive system.

The last stage is the Elimination Stage, from 4:00 a.m. through 12:00 p.m.) At this point, your body has already digested and absorbed the food from the day before. Now it is time to eliminate what the body does not need.

This is not to say that our bodies do not digest, absorb or eliminate at other times of the day, but that these time periods are the most efficient times for those particular bodily functions.

Fruits are the cleansers of the body. When you eat fruit during the Elimination Stage, it helps facilitate the cleansing process. Fruit also has live enzymes in it to help digest itself, freeing up the body's energy that otherwise would have been spent on digestion. Eating fruit takes very little energy to digest. Eating anything other than fruit, like eggs, bacon, cereal, a bagel, takes a *lot* of the body's energy to digest. According to Harvey Diamond, author of "Fit for Life", eating anything other than fruit in the morning also *interrupts* the elimination process. This means that whatever is in your body that needs to be released is going to stay in the colon for a longer amount of time.

The main goal is to get the food in, absorb its nutrients, and get it out. The sooner waste products are released, the better.

This way of eating also gives your body plenty of vitamins and minerals. Fruit has the highest amount of vitamins of any food category. Vegetables have the highest amount of minerals of any food category.

Fruit also gives your body the *healthy* sugar that it needs for energy. Refined (table) sugar is *not* healthy, and is found in foods such as doughnuts and cake. Be aware that even foods like crackers and chips are made with refined sugar. Why? Many food companies put it in their products to make them taste better. Sugar does not add to the fat content of their product, but it is addicting for many people. Another good reason to put sugar in their product is to get people addicted to it! One well-respected holistic nutrition book, "Staying Healthy with Nutrition," has "table sugar" listed in the *drug section*! It also says that if the FDA had known then what they know now about sugar, they probably would not have approved it due to its addictiveness.

Eating fruit in the morning gives your body *healthy* carbs early in the day when your body needs them. Just like a car, fill your tank with fuel at the beginning of the road trip. Carbs are energy. So start your day with *healthy* carbs.

Convenience is yet another benefit of fruit. It is very easy to grab it and go. Apples, bananas, peaches, nectarines, pears, and a handful of grapes or cherries all travel well. However, because fruit is digested faster than other foods, you may need to eat more often. I keep several pieces of fruit in a small cooler and eat it throughout the morning as needed.

Note: *Your body may crave more fruit when you first start eating fruit until noon. The fruit cravings may be a sign that your body is deficient in certain vitamins and minerals. Once your body has gotten enough of those nutrients, the quantity of fruit you crave will usually decrease. It could also be a sign that you may have Candida (yeast infection). If this is the case, you may need to see a nutritionist who can recommend a body cleanse. See Candida section.*

Which fruits to eat? All fruits are great, but they have different qualities. For example, cantaloupe is very high in nutrients and is digested the quickest (in fifteen to twenty minutes). Watermelon is a great detoxifier. Pears have pectin and are great for moving the bowels. Apples have a little bit of many vitamins within them, like a multi-vitamin. Jay Kordich, the Juiceman, refers to apples as the "multivitamin" fruit. Bananas replace lost sugars, electrolytes, and carbs after an exercise session. Did you know that one banana has more electrolytes than a *gallon* of Gatorade? And it isn't filled with coloring, additives, or chemicals! Dates are great for sweetening up a smoothie and are high in calcium. Pineapple has bromelain, which helps the joints. Strawberry seeds have ellagic acid in them which helps improve the immune system, anti-aging, and helps prevent cancer, according to Jay Kordich.

***Note:** *Dried fruits are high in nutrients, yet also very high in calories. Dried fruit is also more difficult to digest than fresh fruit.*

Fruit Digestion

Fruit is digested much more quickly than any other category of food. It is full of enzymes, which speed up the digestion process. Fruit also has a high water content, which not only hydrates your body but also improves digestion. Dried fruits, however, lack water content and therefore take much longer to digest. The skin texture of dried fruits is tough. It takes water from your body to soften it up and then to break it down. Melons such as cantaloupe, watermelon, and honeydew are digested very quickly due to their high water content. Sub-acid fruits such as apples, grapes, peaches, and pears take about thirty to forty-five minutes to digest. Bananas usually take anywhere from forty-five to sixty minutes. Keep digestion times in mind when going about your activities.

Eating only fruit (and purified water) until noon cleanses your body. Drinking coffee can interrupt the cleansing process. If you are a coffee lover, drink it at noon, or try weaning yourself off of it slowly. Replacing coffee with water will not only hydrate you and make you feel better, but it will also improve your health and energy level! The caffeine in coffee has been known to give the body "false" energy. It "borrows" energy, or tricks the body into believing it has more energy than it does. Using this "borrowed" energy taxes the adrenals, making the body "crash" in order to make up for the borrowed energy.

There are acid fruits, sub-acid fruits, and sweet fruits. Although all fruits cleanse the body, the acid fruits (citrus) are the main cleansers of the fruit family. Citrus fruits include oranges, grapefruit, lemons, and limes. Other acid fruits include strawberries and pineapples. Sub-acid fruits include apples, peaches, and pears. Sweet fruits include bananas, raisins, and dried fruits.

2. FOOD COMBINING

Food combining is a way of eating that allows you to eat all types of foods, yet it still allows for proper digestion, freed-up energy, and internal cleansing. Combining your foods properly will make you feel more comfortable, healthier, and lighter.

FOOD COMBINING GUIDELINES

*Eat only fruit until noon, and only on an empty stomach.
*Eat proteins with vegetables only.
*Eat starches (potatoes, rice, pasta, bread) with vegetables only.
*Eat fruit first when eating other foods at the same meal.

Note: *I recommend waiting thirty to sixty minutes after eating fruit before eating other foods.*

Notice that you should not eat proteins with starchy carbohydrates. It takes two different enzymes to digest starches and proteins. If you mix them in the same meal, digestion will be slowed and you will become very tired, just as you do at Thanksgiving dinner. You know the routine. You eat turkey (protein) and mashed potatoes (starchy carb), stuffing (starchy carb), rolls or bread (more starch)…then you eat pumpkin or pecan pie for dessert (starchy carb).

Then you take a nap.

People say that it's the tryptophan (which is an amino acid) in the turkey that makes you sleepy. Yes, tryptophan is a relaxer, but it is *not* what makes you want to fall asleep! Improper food combining is what makes you sleepy. If you don't believe that, eat turkey with mashed potatoes (or some other starchy carb) and see how you feel. See if you feel like going out for a run. On another day, eat turkey with a salad or raw vegetables. I'll bet you will feel lighter and have more energy.

3. PORTION CONTROL

There is an American fascination with "supersizing." The bigger, the better. The bigger the meal, the better the deal. Whatever. Bigger is not always better! Your stomach only has a certain amount of space to hold a meal. After that space is filled, the stomach stretches. When the stomach stretches, digestion cannot keep up. When this happens, excess calories go into storage…yep, *fat* storage. So do not overeat. Eat a normal-sized meal. What *is* a normal sized meal? Most people don't know anymore. They are confused as to what amount of food they should take in.

Ways of eating based on portion control are for people who refuse to change the types of foods they eat. (Someone once told me a long time ago that there are two things people are very protective about: their money and their food. Most people don't want you messing with either one of those.) If you'd like to follow the portion control way of eating, follow the guidelines below.

The 2/3 Rule

The 2/3 Rule involves cutting your meal size down to two thirds of what you currently eat. Going down by a half is a bit depriving to start with, so I recommend 2/3. If you have two or three items on your plate, cut off one third of each item save it for later, or give it to someone else.

The Palm Rule

The Palm Rule means using your hand to measure your portions of protein and carbs. Proteins should be the size of your whole hand in length, width, and thickness. Carbs should be no bigger than the size of your fist. Veggies? You can eat *all* the veggies you want—the more the better—but *without* the butter and sauces, and so on.

The "Veggies First" Rule

This one is self-explanatory. Eat a lot of vegetables *first* (preferably raw or without butter and sauces), then eat your protein.

The "Doggie Bag" Rule

This is used at restaurants. The trick to this is to ask the waiter to bring the doggie bag *before* you eat your meal. Put half of the meal aside in the container, then enjoy the other half.

The 1/2 Rule

This is sharing. Whether you're eating out or at home, share your meal with someone you love. This promotes eating less. Just make sure you both want the same meal.

CARBS, FATS, AND PROTEINS

Carbohydrates, fats, and proteins are all *macronutrients*. Macronutrients are the major nutritional components of what we eat. It is very important to include them all in your "way of eating."

REAL CARBS

Carbs is short for *carbohydrates*. Carbs provide energy for the body and are what the brain uses to function. The low-carb or no-carb diets do tend to work for weight loss, but are difficult to stay on long term. Depriving your body of carbs tends to make you tired and creates brain fog. Our brains cannot function on fats, nor can they function on protein. So unless you want to be brain-dead, eat carbs.

Some people believe that foods like whole grains, brown rice, or spinach pastas are good carbs, but I believe that fresh raw fruits are the best carbohydrates for your body. They have a higher amount of vitamins and minerals and also have a higher water content. For the amount of calories that you are going to consume, eating fruits for *real carbs* are a better bang for your buck!

STARCHES

Starches are often called *complex carbohydrates*. Most people eat starchy carbs at every meal. We are told that starchy carbs give us energy, so we eat more of them. Energy is great, but there is not much nutritional value in starchy carbs. Fruits? Lots of nutritional value. Starchy carbs? They may have some B vitamins that are nutritious, but not near the amount of vitamins and minerals contained in fruit.

Starchy carbs are usually white foods like pasta, bread, rice, or potatoes.

Some refined starches are full of acid-forming minerals and gluten. They are also low in enzymes and most vitamins compared to the vitamins and minerals contained in fruit. According to Douglas Graham, D.C., author of "Nutrition and Athletic Performance," the gluten in most starchy carbs is responsible for forming mucus and congestion, making it harder to breathe. Because starches are cooked before we eat them, the enzymes are killed and vitamins destroyed. Enzymes and vitamins are what are supposed to help our bodies digest food properly.

REAL WAYS OF EATING

The thing that concerns me the most is wheat's addictive potential. Wheat has fifteen different opioids (molecular structures similar to opium). Opium is a narcotic and has addictive and sedating qualities. Because of the various opioids in wheat or starchy carbs, we tend to return to the starches over and over again. I have always loved bread and could never figure out why I always went back for more and more of it. It was almost like I had a bottomless pit for bread. I would eat a slice or two, and then 20-30 minutes later, find myself going back for another slice, or two, or three. Having eaten wheat over the years, I have felt it's addictive effects. It all made sense to me when I read the books "Grain Damage," by Douglas N. Graham, D.C., and The Carbohydrate Addict's Diet" by doctors Rachael and Richard Heller.

There have been times when I got off track in life and turned to starchy carbs. It starts out fine in the beginning. They taste good and are filling. But are they? If you are "sugar sensitive," you may be more prone to becoming addicted to starches. I have found that if I continue to eat starchy carbs, a switch goes off that says "Go!" I can eat starch until I am full, but I don't seem to stay full. My stomach is physically full, but my brain does not acknowledge that it is full when I eat only starchy carbs.

One of my nutrition books, "The Carbohydrate Addict's Diet," states that when we eat only protein at a meal, our body signals our brain that we've had enough protein. Think about it: how many eggs can you eat in one sitting? Or hamburgers? You usually reach a point where enough is enough and you stop.

Fat is the same way. If you eat only fat at a sitting, eventually your body gets to a point where it signals itself to stop. How many avocados can you eat in one sitting? Or butter? Cheese? You usually get to a point where enough is enough; you may feel sick if you eat any more. A switch goes off and you're done.

What about starchy carbs? If you eat *only* starchy carbs at a meal, you think you are full, so you stop. But soon you feel as if you're hungry again. Physically, your body is still digesting the starchy carbs, but it's as if the switch did not go off and the body did not send the signal to your brain. This may not apply to all people, but if you are sugar sensitive there's a possibility that your cravings for carbs may continue.

The solution? Eat real protein with vegetables. Stay away from the wheat, the gluten, the flour, the starchy carbs. Replace the starchy carbs with fruit. Eat fruit only on an empty stomach. You'll get your vitamins, minerals, enzymes, natural sugar, and your energy.

*NOT-SO-REAL CARBS

You probably already know about Not-So-Real carbs like white bread, rice, and pasta. Of course, the cakes, cookies, doughnuts, and candy are definitely No-No carbs! In fact, anything with bread and sugar in it adds fat to your body much more quickly. Some people can metabolize it better than others. The bread quickly turns to sugar as it is digested and then you have double sugar. This makes your insulin peak. It shoots up very quickly, giving you a bit of energy and then quickly drops to a low point, robbing you of energy. This is what you might call a crash-and-burn type food. Refined sugar may give you a shot of energy in the beginning, but will make most people feel low and fatigued shortly afterwards. It's not a quality or reliable source of energy.

Overeating refined sugar can also produce a "sugar hangover." Some people cannot metabolize a large amount of refined sugar (or any food made with table sugar) at once. The body can only digest and use so much sugar or carbs at a time. Whatever is left over will be stored as (you guessed it) fat! After eating too much sugar, one may experience the following symptoms: nausea, bloating, depression, fatigue, and sluggishness of body and/or brain. Dark circles can also appear under the eyes after a refined sugar overload.

So, if you want to get the most reliable energy, sustained energy, quality energy—*real* energy—eat fresh fruit.

FATS

Fat is a macronutrient that stirs up mixed emotions for most people. Fats are necessary for the body to function; they help "oil" the body. You put oil in your car to make it run more smoothly, and your body needs oil too: food oils.

REAL FATS

Real fats are natural fats. *Real fats* come from *real foods*. These include avocados, flaxseed oil, olive oil, coconut oil, and so on. Some fruits and vegetables have a very small amount of real fat that is healthy for the body. In fact, the *real fats* can help your body lose weight and get rid of excess body fat! Your body has brown fat and white fat. Brown fat, or brown adipose tissue, is the fat that is essential for your body to function. This fat is associated with body temperature and keeping the body warm. It also has more capillaries than white fat (or white adipose tissue.) White fat is excess fat: the fat most people don't want. Avocados, a monounsaturated fat, are high in fat, but they are considered a healthy fat which helps raise your metabolism, thereby helping you to lose unwanted weight. Avocados help your body get rid of the white fat! So don't think that all fats are bad. *Real fats* are good fats!

NOT-SO-REAL FATS

Cream, butter, sour cream, and foods made with hydrogenated oils (such as processed food), are foods that contain the kind of fats we should avoid. These *Not-So Real fats* are those that are cooked at high temperatures. Once these fats are cooked, it changes the molecular structure and they enter your body as trans fats. Trans fats are No-No fats. Step away from any food that is labeled as containing hydrogenated oils or partially hydrogenated oils. They are very unhealthy. These are the fats that make your body fatter and fatter. These dangerous fats clog your arteries.

PROTEINS

Real proteins are protein-rich foods with a low amount of fat—such as most dried beans, fish, turkey, chicken, raw nuts, and seeds. Once again, when proteins are also fried, trans fatty acids are created, making them harmful to the body. For better health, please, *no* fried proteins!

FALLING OFF TRACK

We have all done it: fallen off track. You know. You've had the "maybe just one bite won't hurt" thought. Then forty-five bites later, you've realized you've gone off track from your *real healthy* way of eating.

Maybe something negative happens in your life that you have no control over—maybe a loved one is suddenly gone from your life. So, you throw everything out the window, except what you feel. That's all that matters at the time: the way you feel.

You don't care about how healthy you had been eating or how good you were feeling. Something happens, you put life on hold, and all bets are off. Time and life just stop. You need to feel.

Now, you don't want to feel the pain, but you must. If you don't feel the pain, you will try to numb it, do anything you can to escape it and not to feel it. When I lost my mother in 2009, I tried to numb my pain with starchy carbs, overeating, alcohol, and yes, smoking...the big taboo. I felt that as long as I was doing at least one of these things, I was escaping the pain. It didn't work, but I didn't care. I hurt so badly at the time that I didn't care if it all killed me, because then I would not be feeling the pain. I thought it would be great if the unhealthy food, alcohol, and cigarettes killed me, because then I could join my mother in heaven and not feel any emotional pain.

In fact, typing this is bringing up emotions about my mother right now. But as I type, I realize how therapeutic writing is. When we are experiencing a traumatic event in our life, however, we don't normally think to pick up a pen and start writing away the pain. In the past, I would eat, drink, or smoke as stressful events would come up and only years later did I think about better tools for releasing the pain. Don't get me wrong, I am not perfect, none of us are. I know I "should" be doing yoga or journaling when I am hurt, stressed out, or in pain, but the last thing I tend to think of when I am in crisis is doing a yogic tree pose or looking for my pen and journal. When stressed or in pain, we tend to grab what is easiest and quickest—which usually tends to be food, cigarettes, or alcohol. And we tend to go for foods that give us comfort: usually the soft, creamy types of foods, like macaroni and cheese or ice cream.

So we binge, feel terrible, and then realize that it did not make us feel good—or not for very long, anyway—and then we decide to get back on track, because deep down we do want to feel good. And even though we get off track for a while and many of us tend to beat ourselves up about it, it still feels good for those few moments when you finally bite into that mac'n cheese you hadn't had in five months. So, although it is not a long term solution to healing your body, mind, and heart, at least you did get some "soul" food for a moment.

CANDIDA

Candida is one reason people get off track. While working at an internal health clinic, I learned that Candida is yeast growth within the body. It can grow in many different areas of the body, such as the mouth, the vagina, the colon—even the brain! We always have some amount of yeast in our bodies. When the amount of yeast gets out of balance, that's when the problems start. Candida, or yeast overgrowth, can be caused by eating too much bread or yeast-filled foods, sugar, and/or alcohol. These types of foods and drink tend to feed the Candida and make it grow. Once it gets to a certain point of overgrowth, it can be very difficult to resist cravings for these foods.

There are a couple of ways to reduce the yeast overgrowth, or at least control it. One way is to go on a Candida diet. Such diets usually consist of vegetables and proteins only; no fruit, bread, alcohol or sugars. When I was a raw foodist, I heard that eating only pineapple for an extended amount of time would do the trick. I never did try it, but I heard that the acid in the pineapple helps kill the excess yeast growth.

Proper food combining helps prevent Candida; however, I believe the best way to rid myself of Candida was by using a Rife machine or frequency generator. (See section on Holistic Machines). The Rife machine is a frequency generator that has a Candida frequency. You punch in the Candida frequency code then hold the two cylindrical metal handles for forty-seven minutes while the electrical frequency zaps the negative microorganisms. Once the Candida/yeast growth is back in balance, you should be okay. Make sure you drink a large glass of water after the Rife session. Drinking water helps to flush out the "die-off," or toxins.

If you continue to eat breads and yeast-filled foods, excessive sugar, and/or alcohol, then you may need to use the Rife machine on a regular basis. I usually do one or two sessions per week for maintenance, or more if I have gotten off track with my eating.

BINGEING

Bingeing is overeating: eating when we are not hungry or do not stop after our stomach is full. We usually do this when we are upset, bored, or in emotional pain. I know; I have done it many times.

There have been times when I knew I was not hungry anymore, yet still continued to eat. I have eaten so much at a sitting that my stomach hurt. It was as if I was trying to put food down my body in order to stop the feelings from coming up. I could feel emotion bubbling up inside of me, yet was fearful of what it was and how to cope with it. Instead of feeling the emotional pain, I tried to numb it by comforting myself with food. Alcohol and drugs are not the only way to escape our feelings; bingeing also numbs us. It is better to release the feelings, cry it out, scream, hit a pillow, or write out the feelings through journaling. Trying to go around the pain does not work. Going *through* the pain does work.

Overeating puts something *into* our bodies when really, something needs to *come out*. The feelings need to come out; otherwise, they stay inside and continue to cause pain. Over time, the pain gets worse and the problem continues, as does the bingeing.

So, next time you feel some emotion coming up...let it come. Let the feelings come up and let them out. Release the feelings and emotion in a way that frees you. You may feel better after writing the feelings out in a journal. You may feel better after crying. Or you may journal and cry. Whatever works for you, get it out. Don't put something in your body. Let it out.

After the bingeing, there's the guilt. It makes the experience worse if you beat yourself up. Remember, we are human, not perfect. Remember that perfection is fake and artificial, not *real*. I say acknowledge the feelings, face them, and let them go. Once you have let the feelings go, you will be ready to get back on track. When you reach the point where you have cried it all out, written it out, or screamed it out, then, you'll be at peace. Then you'll be ready to get back on track.

Congratulate yourself for letting it go and getting back on track.

Thought-Less/Association Eating: Things that tend to make us engage in unnecessary eating.

TELEVISION

We tend to eat *more* while watching TV and do not pay attention to:

* What we are doing
* What we are eating
* What the food tastes like
* What it smells like
* What it looks like

We eat more because we are in a "television trance." Also, commercials on television tend to make us want to eat when we're not really hungry. Turn the TV off. Play some music. Read a book.

Thirst

We tend to eat when, really, we are just thirsty. Next time you are hungry, drink eight to twelve ounces of water. Wait ten or fifteen minutes. If you are still hungry, then eat. If you're not, you never were to begin with.

Tiredness

We tend to eat when we are feeling fatigued. We reach for food thinking that the food will give us energy, when really, what we need is sleep. Put the food down. Take a nap.

Triggers

Some of us enter our homes through the kitchen and subconsciously respond to being there by reaching for food. Try using a different entrance. Or, get in the habit of doing something else after entering, like lighting a candle, putting on some music, or other activity.

Reading

We tend to eat more while reading. Set the book down. Enjoy your food.

Lack of Human touch

We tend to eat more when we lack human touch. Give someone a hug. Cuddle with someone. If you are single or in need of human touch, buy yourself a massage. You deserve it. Or *give* a massage; someone will love you for it.

GETTING BACK ON TRACK

You come to a point where you've decided to get back on track. You are ready to start feeling good, or better. You are ready to start eating healthy again, because you remember how good you felt. You felt lean, strong, and healthy when you were eating *real health* foods. You felt light, energetic, positive and happy. You know that this is how you are supposed to feel. So eat fruit until noon, eat protein with veggies, and start feeling *real health* again.

It's much tougher to get back on track after you've fallen off. So, be proud of yourself for getting back at it! People are respected more for picking themselves up and getting back on track than someone who plods along, never improving themselves.

You have reached way down inside yourself, gotten **real** and honest with yourself and decided to get back to where you feel best—back on track! Give yourself a compliment, hot bath, massage, something to reward yourself for your strength and courage.

Thought-Full Eating: A few tips to exchange thought-less eating for thought-full eating:

LOOK at your food

SMELL your food

FEEL your food

TASTE your food. Really taste and savor it.

EAT only when you are truly hungry. Listen to that incredible body of yours. If you really listen, it will speak to you.

FOOD SENSITIVITIES

Food sensitivities can be a frustrating thing to deal with. There are ways around them if you know what foods you are sensitive to. The allergist I once worked for recommended an elimination diet which involves eliminating eight different food categories for five days. These categories include: eggs, grains, dark sodas, sugar, dairy, citrus fruits and juices, tomatoes, and yes, chocolate. Hey, it's only for five days! After the fifth day, you can add the food that you missed most back into your diet. What you *can* eat is: fruit (non-citrus), vegetables (no tomatoes), fish, turkey, chicken, beef, and water (woo-hoo!).

When you start adding the food you missed most back into your diet, make sure you pay attention to how you feel and how your body reacts. Symptoms can include headaches, a stuffed-up or runny nose, throat-clearing of mucus, fatigue and many others. To get more information on food allergies and the elimination diet, read Dr. Russell Roby's book, *Maybe It IS All in Your Head…And You Are NOT Crazy.*

* * *

SECTION II:

REAL HEALTH: PHYSICAL & ENVIRONMENTAL

REAL EXERCISE

Real exercise is moving your body in a natural and healthy way. If you perform any type of activity that does not feel natural or healthy, stop doing it. *Real exercise* makes your blood pump. The blood carries nutrients from the *real food* you eat to all of the necessary organs. The body absorbs those nutrients, resulting in a *real body* with *real health*. Exercise can also speed the healing of some injuries. Exercise helps pump blood, which carries nutrients to the injury site within the body, thereby helping the injury heal quicker.

Real exercise is also enjoyable. Find a type of exercise that makes you feel good. Studies have shown that when people participate in exercises that they enjoy, they are more likely to stick with them.

Real exercise is beneficial to the body at almost any time of day. Exercising in the morning helps wake your body up and helps you think more clearly. Studies have shown that morning exercisers are also more likely to stick with their exercise program. If you're not a morning person, don't let that stop you. If you are an afternoon or early evening exerciser, go for it. Any exercise at any time is a good thing. However, because exercise stimulates the adrenaline in your body, exercising too late at night can cause sleep difficulties.

Always make sure you do a ten minute warm-up before exercising.

2-WAY EXERCISE

2-Way Exercise is a program that I have designed to work your body and your brain. 2-Way Exercise works you physically and mentally.

Real Physical Exercise includes cardio and weight-bearing exercise. Cardiovascular exercise (or *cardio*) creates *real health* for your cardiovascular system. Weight-bearing exercises create *real health* for your bones and muscular system.

Real Cardio (exercise that helps improve the health of the heart and lungs) creates *real health* by pumping blood, improving lung capacity and strengthening your heart. Some examples of *real cardio* are aerobics, cycling, race walking, running, hiking, or kickboxing.

Real Weight-Bearing Exercise creates a stronger skeletal system through better bone density. The impact of the weight on your bones compacts the bone tissue. Once the bone tissues are compacted, the bones become denser and stronger. *Real weight-bearing exercise* also strengthens your muscular system. The weight of your body or exercise weights that you lift increase the strength of your muscles and bones. Any type of exercise that includes weights, and/or your own body weight and the resistance of gravity are considered weight-bearing exercise. Examples of weight-bearing exercises that use your own body weight are running, jumping, pushups, lunges, squats, tricep dips, etc.

Strength training can be done with free weights, weight machines, resistance bands or tubing, and stability balls. These types of exercises create strength as muscles work against weight and the pull of gravity.

REAL MENTAL EXERCISE

The other component to 2-Way Exercise, *real mental exercise*, is about exercising your brain while you exercise your body. I am not talking about reading a book or magazine while you sit on a stationary bike. *Real mental exercise* is a way of empowering your mind, your self-esteem, and your confidence as well as your body. *A strong mind creates a strong body; whatever starts in the mind, the body follows.*

So, to create a strong mind, start talking. Tell your incredible body how strong it is. Tell it how powerful it is, how healthy it is, how lean it is, how fast it is. Tell it anything and everything that is positive and healthy. Tell it and it will become it.

Even if you don't believe what you're saying at first, keep it up. You will reprogram your way of thinking. Your brain will get used to hearing and thinking those powerful words and will start to believe them. Once your brain hears it, thinks it, and believes it...your body will *become* it.

If you are on the treadmill running, you will develop a rhythm. As you run, come up with a mantra. Something like "I am lean, strong, and healthy...I am lean, strong, and healthy...I am lean, strong, and healthy. Say something that fits you and your goals, over and over again. As you say your mantra, it will flow right into the rhythm. This not only empowers your brain and your body, but it also makes the time on the treadmill go by quickly.

If you are lifting weights in front of a mirror, pick five to ten different affirmations about yourself and your goals. What is it you want to be? It must be positive and healthy. This is like healthy food for your brain, mind, and self-esteem. Instead of counting repetitions when lifting weights, affirm yourself. Affirm your health, your strength, your, power, and so on. You can even go into intangibles like success, honesty, or commitment.

Here is an example of what to say during weight lifting. You can say an affirmation at each repetition. The group below is used over five reps. Say it twice and you've got ten reps…three times and you've got fifteen reps.

Rep #1   "I am Lean"
Rep #2   "I am Strong"
Rep #3   "I am Healthy"
Rep #4   "I am Successful"
Rep #5   "I am Wealthy"

Make sure you say "I am" at the beginning of each affirmation and that your words are positive and healthy. Remember: don't tell yourself what you *don't* want to be. Tell yourself what you *do* want to be!

Tip: If you can, look yourself in the left eye as you say these affirmations.If you are in a crowded gym and are feeling a bit self-conscious, you can still say the affirmations to yourself quietly. Forming the words and hearing them while thinking the thoughts will make an impact on your brain and your body.

Remember, anytime you say or even think a negative thought about your body or self, your brain records it. Each time your brain hears or thinks that negative thought, it makes a stronger and stronger imprint in your brain. The neurons in your brain brand that thought stronger and deeper each time you think it or say it.

The same goes for positive, healthy talk. Tell your incredible self that you are intelligent, strong, and healthy, and the neurons will make that imprint on your brain stronger and deeper each time you say it and think it.

Think strong. Talk strong. BE strong.

CORE COMPONENTS OF REAL FITNESS

The core components of *Real Fitness* are strength, speed, and endurance.

Strength Training: Creating muscle strength is the first component of Real Fitness. You know it...weights, free weights, or weight machines; bands or tubing, stability ball, and so forth.

Speed (Cardio): So, your body is strong, but is it fast? The best way I know to create speed is to run on a treadmill or outside. Other ways to create speed are cycling, elliptical machine, etc. To create speed, make sure you do interval training.

Endurance: Your body is strong and fast, but for how *long*, is it strong and fast? You already have the strength, and speed; now create the endurance. Lift the weight and hold it for a long time, doing very slow repetitions.

The goal of Real Fitness is to have all three components; strength, speed, and endurance.

REAL CARDIO

INTERVAL TRAINING

Interval training is a cardio technique to increase a person's fitness level and speed up the metabolism by increasing the workload over and above what the body is normally used to. This results in increased calorie burn. Interval training increases the heart rate for a certain amount of time, then brings the heart rate back down to a moderate level to recover, but not to fully cool down. The amount of time to increase the heart rate can be anything from ten seconds to four-to five minute intervals and will depend on the fitness level of the individual. A speed interval can be a ten-second sprint on a bike or a one-minute sprint on a treadmill. Some people start out with ten-second intervals, then move to fifteen, thirty, and forty-five seconds, and then up to one minute.

Intervals can be done back to back, increasing speed or intensity with each interval, or recovery time can be placed between them. It all depends on what state of health you are in and what you are capable of doing. If you have any heart issues or physical limitations, you may want to exclude interval training from your workout schedule, since interval training can be hard on the body. If pushed too hard, the body can be worn down and the immune system compromised.

Please get approval from your healthcare practitioner before taking part in interval training.

KICKBOXING

This is not only a calorie burner, but also educational. It usually involves moves from martial arts, self-defense, and sometimes added aerobic or cross-training exercises. Some of kickboxing's basic moves are jabs, hooks, uppercuts, knee cocks, kicks (front, side and rear kicks), knee slams, and elbow jabs.

For safety reasons, it is important that you have a certified kickboxing instructor. The sport can be very intense, but only if you make it that way. Be sure to use proper form, since its quick, intense movements can cause injury if not performed properly. Make sure your arms and legs extend no more than 95 percent of the way out. This will help you use more muscle, burn more calories and prevent you from snapping the joints (knees, elbows and shoulders).

There's a good chance you'll sweat when you kickbox. It may take a few classes to get the moves, but once you get the basics down, you'll be in for a great workout. The beauty of kickboxing is that it works both upper and lower body. You can burn up to seven hundred calories per hour depending on how much intensity you put into the moves.

NIA DANCE

NIA stands for Non-impact Integrated Aerobics— NIA is more than just low-impact dancing. It is movement that not only frees the body, but also frees the mind.

You may feel a bit silly doing the moves at first, but once you realize that no one is watching, you can let go and feel free to express yourself. Usually everyone else in the class is busy dancing and moving in their own NIA world. There is no right or wrong way to do it. It is instructor guided, but there is freedom in the way you choose to express the movements. NIA dance is a good cardio workout, therapeutic and great for relieving stress.

CROSS-TRAINING

Cross-training means to "cross" over into other exercises besides the exercises your body is used to doing. It is a combination of strength training and cardio exercises. Cross-training helps to strengthen all different muscles in all different ways. This variety of exercise helps to train your body in ways it is not used to. When cross-training, the muscles will adapt and expand into a stronger and more varied form of training.

For example, someone who runs on a regular basis is performing linear movement. The muscles adapt to moving forward over and over again. This adaptation is good exercise for the body, but it can also make trying out a new form of exercise more dangerous. When the muscles are used to linear movement only, they are not yet trained or strengthened laterally. If this runner tries a new form of exercise like rollerblading, the lateral movements which the muscles are not used to doing could increase the likelihood of injury. If one cross-trains on a regular basis, muscles used to a variety of movements are more likely to hold up during new exercises.

Overall, cross-training helps give your body a well-rounded level of fitness. Mix up your exercise routine. *Make it a routine to get out of a routine.* Do a variety of exercises and see your body's fitness level improve.

BOOT CAMPS

"Boot camp" classes have become very popular over the last few years. They can be experienced indoors or outdoors, and usually include a variety of strength training and cardio exercises. Some boot camps may include military style exercises. These can include lunges and squats, running, jumping jacks, push-ups, and other calisthenics.

Some boot camps include interval training. The goal for most boot-campers is to get an intense workout in a short amount of time.

REBOUNDING/MINI-TRAMPOLINE

Rebounding is the best all-around exercise and a fun and effective way to get your body in shape. It was invented in 1936 and introduced to the armed services prior to World War II. It was used to develop balance, dexterity, coordination, rhythm, and timing. It improved strength and fitness.

Rebounding stimulates the neuromuscular system in ways that can be achieved with no other exercise. It combines gravity, acceleration, and deceleration. According to Dr. Hans Gruenn, alternating weightlessness and increased gravitational pull (or G force) exercises every single cell, organ, and muscle. The rebound workout is also great for the body's joints. Bouncing on the rebounder removes the hard surface used when running, doing aerobics, or any other land exercise. The rebounder absorbs the shock of the joints, allowing the body to work harder and longer. People with joint problems embrace this piece of equipment because it helps to make exercising pain-free. According to Harvey Diamond, author of "Fit for Life II," even people in wheelchairs can benefit from the rebounder by placing their feet on the rebounder as someone else jumps on it.

While acquiring my rebounding certification, I learned that rebounding also has detoxifying capabilities. Since your lymphatic system does not have a pump, the gravity/pressure from jumping acts as one. This "pumping" cleanses your lymphatic system and helps to detoxify your body. Bouncing a minimum of five to ten minutes can help just about anyone loosen up toxins to be eliminated from the body.

The way you jump matters. Jumping high is fun, but it is not the most effective workout. As you jump, press downward. Pretend there is a low ceiling above your head. Putting your body weight into the downward motion creates a more challenging workout and helps to improve your overall fitness. If you're not into an effective or intense workout, regular jumping is also beneficial. Your body still receives exercise, your lymphatic system still pumps out toxins, and you have fun!

Whether you have stiff joints or not, try the rebounder. It will give your body exercise, improve your health, and make you feel like a kid again! When I jump on the rebounder, it reminds me of jumping up and down on Mom and Dad's bed as a child.

*Note: *If you need to release pressure or clear up your nasal passages, try bouncing on the rebounder for a minimum of five minutes. The vertical bouncing pumps your lymphatic system to help you breathe better!* ***Also,*** *those with bladder issues may experience some leakage at first, but with practice, rebounding can strengthen the muscles within the bladder!*

Benefits of Rebounding:

* Builds muscle
* Strengthens heart
* Strengthens joints
* Improves posture
* Improves coordination

* Helps improve metabolism
* Improves digestion
* Improves elimination
* Corrects poor eyesight
* Stimulates lymph system (helps detox your body)

* Circulates more oxygen to tissues

* Improves body alignment

* Adds flexibility to neck, knees, hips, ankles, and back

The rebounder is cleansing, healthy, and fun! Try the rebounder for your next workout and feel the difference!

WATER FITNESS

Movement in water is a great way to strength train. The resistance of movement under water is twelve times the resistance of movement against air. When exercising on land, gravity takes over on the down movement. Water can provide equal resistance in both directions. With water, the harder you resist the water, the tougher the workout.

Adding water "toys" such as water weights, water noodles, and kickboards can also create variety in your workout. If it's too hot to exercise or you're bored with your regular workout, try making a splash with water fitness!

REAL STRENGTH
TRAINING
(Reproduced as Handout
in Appendix)

BENEFITS:

*Strengthens bones

*Strengthens muscles

*Strengthens connective tissue

*Improves physical ability

*Prevents injuries

*Increases metabolism

GUIDELINES:

*Start with a warm-up to increase body temperature (walking, marching).

*8–12 repetitions with weights that are somewhat challenging.

*3 sets if time allows. If not, do 1 set(1 set gives you 92 percent of the benefits of doing 3 sets)

*Start with large muscle groups (legs, chest, back, glutes/buttocks), then move to small muscle groups (shoulders, biceps, triceps).

*Move weight with a 95 percent range of motion.

*Exhale on the exertion part of the movement. (Blow out on the hard part of exercise.)

*Slower is better. Slower is more challenging. Slower is more effective. Slower is safer.

*Give muscles forty-eight hours rest between workout sessions

*End your workout with stretches, or stretch the muscles worked between each set. Hold each stretch for at least ten seconds or longer. This allows oxygen to get in and rebuilds the muscles better and stronger.

RECOMMENDED STRENGTH TRAINING EXERCISES:

Exercise	Muscle Group
Leg Press	Quads, Glutes - front thighs and butt
Leg Curl	Hamstrings – back of thighs
Chest Press	Pectorals - chest
Lat Pull Down	Lats - back
Row	Trapezius – upper back
Overhead Press	Deltoids - shoulders
Overhead Extension	Triceps – upper back arms
Arm Curl	Biceps – front upper arms
Crunches	Abdominals – stomach/ribcage area
Back Extension	Erector Spinae - back

STABILITY BALL

This big rubber ball, which is similar to a beach ball, has become extremely popular. It was first used in physical therapy clinics to help post-surgery and post-injury patients regain their muscle strength and balance. It can be used to improve stability and balance and also in stretching and strength training. Many people and offices have replaced their desk chairs with the stability ball. Sitting upright on it can improve your core muscles: back, oblique and abdominal muscles.

Most people use the ball for doing abdominal or core exercises, but there is so much more to do with this basic, inexpensive tool. Try taking a ball class. In other words, "have a ball" on the ball! Hand weights can also be incorporated into your stability ball workout to mix up your normal workout routine. (See Appendix for Stability Ball handout)

RESISTANCE BANDS

Resistance bands are an inexpensive, convenient way to increase strength or tone your body. They are similar to large rubber bands that are lightweight and easy to store or travel with. Resistance bands are also a great way to supplement your weight workout.

Benefits of Resistance Bands
*Free range of movement
*Various speeds of movement
*Lightweight
*Easy to travel with
*Easy to store
*Great for injury rehabilitation
*Improve muscle strength
*Increase muscle size
*Lower body fat

REAL CORE

Core conditioning is about strengthening the abdominal, back, obliques and gluteus muscles (buttocks). When your core muscles are strong, you are less likely to get injured and also create a stable center within your body. Consider a tree and its trunk. That's like your core. When you have a strong trunk, the trunk is then better able to lift and hold up the branches (your arms and legs). A stronger core helps to prevent back problems. When conditioning and strengthening your core, make sure you strengthen the core from all sides. Include exercises for the upper abs, lower abs, internal obliques (muscles along the side of your waist), external obliques (muscles along the front of your ribs cage, right/left side), rectus abdominus and the upper and lower back.

To protect your back/core, keep these things in mind:

*A proper warm-up and cool-down before and after flexibility exercises is very important.

*Maintain a healthy weight. This decreases strain on your back.

*Sit upright on a stability ball to improve posture. You can use one in place of a computer chair.

*Sleep on a firm mattress. Try sleeping on your back with a pillow under your knees to relieve unnecessary pressure on the lower back.

*Use leg muscles to do most of the work when lifting. (Bend at knees, not waist.)

*Do not stand in one position for too long. Shift body weight from leg to leg.

*Do not sit for long periods of time. Stand and stretch every thirty to sixty minutes.

*Try to avoid emotional stress (yeah, right!) Emotional stress causes muscle tension.

STABILITY BALL

The stability ball is used for abdominal/core exercises. This versatile piece of equipment helps strengthen the upper and lower abs as well as the internal and external obliques. The ball can also be used to strengthen the back in a variety of different exercises. . (See Appendix for Stability Ball handout)

MORE CORE...

Mechanical bull machines, popularized by the 1980 movie, *Urban Cowboy*, simulate the motion of what cowboys experience in rodeo bull riding. This motion of "bull riding" works the upper and lower abs as well as the internal and external obliques. This workout can also help strengthen the back and inner thighs while making the workout unique and fun!

Note: This activity is not recommended for those with neck or back issues.

REAL STRETCHING

FLEXIBILITY/STRETCHING & OXYGENATING OUR MUSCLES

People in the exercise industry have always told me it was important to stretch, but they never explained *why* it was important to stretch. So, guess what? I never really stretched much. I didn't think it was that important. But it is. If I understand the importance of doing something, I'll do it.

Flexibility is important for increasing range of motion and oxygenating muscle. Range of motion is needed when reaching for things. As we age, flexibility and range of motion decreases. The simple act of reaching for an item on the shelf can become a major effort.

Before performing any type of stretch or exercise, please be sure to warm your muscles up. March in place. Move your arms, legs, and body in a rhythmic motion for at least five to ten minutes before performing your stretches. Why? It will help prevent injury. Imagine your muscles being like taffy. If you put a piece of taffy in the freezer and then apply pressure to it, it will snap or break. If you heat a piece of taffy in the microwave, and then apply pressure, it will stretch and stretch and stretch. Get the idea? Muscles need to be warm before stretching.

Whenever we stretch, we oxygenate our muscles. Why is that important? Well, it makes the muscles stronger. If you stretch your muscles and hold the stretch for at least ten seconds, you will allow oxygen into your muscles. Most people hold their stretches for only four or five seconds. That is not long enough. When you apply pressure to the muscle (the act of stretching), the muscle initially tightens up. That is called the *stretch reflex*. The muscle thinks that it is going to be injured. Once you hold the stretch for a while, the muscle starts to relax. It realizes that it is not going to be injured. That's when the oxygen gets into the muscle to rebuild it better and stronger. So make your stretching worthwhile. Hold those stretches for at least ten seconds!

Another good reason to oxygenate the muscles is to help avoid cancer. According to the article "Understanding Cancer and Cancer Cells, cancer cells cannot survive in an environment where there is oxygen. Oxygenate your muscles. Stretch like a cat. Stretch like a dancer. Stretch like taffy. Just stretch!

Cats stretch their muscles every day—several times a day, in fact, Because of this, cats are sleek and agile. Stretching your muscles can create sleeker, longer muscles. If you don't like cats, think of dancers. Dancers are always stretching. What are their bodies and muscles like? Their bodies are long, sleek and healthy. One way to create long, sleek, healthy muscles is to do basic stretches for five to ten minutes every day.

Stretching on a regular basis helps to achieve balance in flexibility. Flexibility balance is when the front and back of your body, as well as right and left sides, are equally flexible. Balance in flexibility helps improve posture and reduce the likelihood of injury.

Flexibility can be improved in just five to twenty minutes a day. Whatever you do, make sure you stretch at least once a week! Flexibility can be lost after a week.

SERENITY STRETCH

Regular stretching can be boring. In fact, that's one reason why many people don't do it. Another reason is that they don't understand its importance. Make stretching relaxing and enjoyable by doing Serenity Stretch. It is lengthening and elongating the muscles while listening to soothing music, ending with a relaxing, seven- to ten-minute meditation. Serenity Stretch is an *experience*.

YOGA

Yoga is hot these days and seems to keep growing in popularity. There are many types of yoga, including the classic hatha yoga, ashtanga, vinyasa, and bikram styles.

Yoga is about stretching, flexibility, strengthening, improving posture, body awareness, breathing, and centering. People do yoga for different reasons. One person may enjoy the flexibility it provides to tight muscles, while another may seek its inner peace and centering aspects. No matter what reason you do it, it can offer many more benefits than you may be aware of.

Benefits of Yoga

The benefits of yoga include internal benefits as well as external benefits. Emotional, physical, and general health benefits are some to consider as well as disease prevention. Some of the things that yoga has been known to help:

*Reduce blood pressure   *Decrease heart rate
*Improve mood   *Decrease stress
*Improve circulation   *Improve focus and
*Improve muscle tone   concentration

*Strengthen immune system

*Improve digestion

*Massage internal organs

*Detoxify the body

*Improve balance

*Improve sleep

*Improve posture

*Increase energy

*Decrease cholesterol

*Strengthen lymphatic system

*Improve breathing

*Improve carpal tunnel syndrome

*Improve constipation

*Help prevent cancer

*Increase calmness

*Help lift depression

*Decrease anxiety

*Reduce oxygen needs

*Decrease likelihood of injury

*Increase well-being

*Increase strength

*Balance normal body weight

*Balance flexibility within body

*Help prevent osteoporosis

*Improve range of motion

*Decrease migraines

*Improve asthma

*Improve back pain

REAL BALANCE

Balance is very important but is often taken for granted. You cannot do anything without balance—you can't stand, walk, or even sit up. If we don't balance well, we don't function well. Balance becomes more and more important as we age. Elderly people can prevent falls and injuries by improving their balance.

You can create *real balance* through exercises without equipment or you can choose from many balance tools. Practice balancing on equipment such as a Bosu, a wobble board, or a stability ball. If you're not into equipment or gadgets, do balance exercises like standing on one leg.

Practicing yoga is a popular way to improve balance. Tree pose and triangle pose are particularly helpful, as are many other asanas (poses). Check out your local yoga studio or buy one of the many good instructional DVDs and learn to do yoga in the privacy of your own home. Some I have used and enjoyed are by Rodney Yee. Another beautifully done yoga DVD is by Ali McGraw.

BOSU

The Bosu is a piece of equipment that looks like half of a stability ball. One side is flat, hard plastic and the other side is rubber, dome-shaped, and filled with air. It is a versatile piece of equipment that can improve your balance and create variety in your workout.

The Bosu was originally designed to improve balance by strengthening the stabilizing muscles. Balance exercises can be performed on either side of the Bosu. The flat side can be used for surfer-style balancing, while the dome-shaped side can be used to practice balance while jumping. It strengthens the ankles, legs, and core of the body. The Bosu can also be used for cardio and a variety of strength training exercises.

FALLING OFF TRACK

Just as we can get off track with our eating, we can do the same with exercise.

When I found out that my boyfriend was sleeping with his ex-girlfriend, all bets were off. One of the ways I tried numbing the pain was by eating very little food. Being that stressed, I stopped exercising and had no appetite. I felt as if I was escaping the pain. It didn't work, but I didn't care. If it killed me, I would not be feeling the pain and feeling like a failure. I felt a sense of inadequacy, as if I had done something wrong or was not good enough. After all the time and energy I spent trying to make my body perfect! Still, not perfect?

This had never happened before. Was I not pretty enough? Was my body not young enough, lean enough, or sexy enough? We had a great sex life, so what was wrong with me? I was harming my health, but I didn't care. At the time, subconsciously, I just wanted to hurt myself, because I felt that I was not good enough. Not perfect.

Was I expected to be perfect in an imperfect world? Did I choose someone to be in a relationship that expected perfection? Or was *I* so focused on being perfect that I attracted someone who also expected perfection from me?

Let me tell you, perfectionism is a tough order to fill. Actually, it's exhausting, and you never get there. When we feel we are striving for the perfect body, that's when we need to check in with ourselves and be *real*. It's time to take a look at ourselves and decide what we are and what we are not.

Maybe this was an opportunity to learn something about myself— to go deep within, look at what I was, and consider what I could be. Or, maybe my partner was the one who had serious issues to resolve.

It can all be so confusing while it is happening. We tend to stop, throw out all "healthy" ideas and focus on the question "Why is this happening?" It's never easy to get the answer while something is actually happening to you. The answer does seem to come most times—but later, after we've gotten through it. Then it makes sense. Then we understand. And then, maybe we will even be grateful that it happened because it made us a better, stronger, and wiser person.

When things that challenge us happen and we don't understand, it drives us crazy. I felt like I wanted an answer, right then. But the answer didn't come that day; it took time—which allowed me to ask, "What am I to learn from this?"

I've found over the years that letting an event destroy me makes me a powerless victim.

Now, when negative things happen, I ask myself, "What am I supposed to learn from this?" I am *not* saying that we should be doormats and take all kinds of abuse from people and life. I *am* saying that none of us are perfect—not our friends, our lovers, our partners, and not us. We *all* have things to learn from our situations.

I will tell you that after the worst was over, I decided to look at the silver lining in that black cloud (yes, it felt very black at the time).

First, I decided early on that at least I had experienced what it felt like to be in this situation. I had seen so many depressing Lifetime movies over the years when I used to watch television. When infidelity happened to me, I felt as if I were like a victim in a movie. But, more importantly, I now know how other people feel. Instead of remaining a victim, I chose to use the experience as a way to understand people, to connect with and to relate to those who had been through it. I have turned this negative experience into a healing tool.

The second piece of silver lining was that the experience made me reach deep down inside and see some things I hadn't seen before. I saw some things about myself that I didn't like and did not want to face the truth. I took these ugly truths and began to work on them. I became a person of self-growth: someone who was willing to take a look at myself, for *real*.

I now feel stronger and more understanding of others in similar situations. I feel I am a better person because of it.

In no way do I condone the behavior of infidelity, but I do recognize that there are all kinds of pain and all kinds of ways that people deal with it.

The goal is for us to learn from our mistakes and move on. Don't beat yourself up. After the other person has apologized authentically, forgive them. Set yourself free from the pain, take it as a learning experience, and move on as a better, more well-rounded person. Take the path of most light. Taking actions of darkness keeps you in darkness. Taking the higher path leads you to higher ground, releases the pain, and moves you forward.

I now think of my body as strong, healthy, and functional. Instead of focusing on its imperfections, I focus on how amazing it is that it performs all of its functions every day—whether walking, standing, breathing, digesting, singing, dancing, or being able to see the beauty of nature.

Your body is an amazing organism.

Appreciate it.

Learn from it.

Know full well that you are getting back on track, and…

Congratulate yourself for getting back on track.

GETTING BACK ON TRACK

This is the point where you've decided to get back on track. You are ready to start exercising again, because you remember how good you felt. You felt lean, strong, and healthy when you were exercising. You felt light, energetic, positive, and happy. So get on the treadmill, or bounce your way back into exercise by jumping on a rebounder. Whether it is doing strength training or going for a daily walk, do your body a favor and start feeling *real health* again.

Feel good about yourself for having the strength to get back on track. It's much tougher to get back on track after you've fallen off. So, be proud of yourself for getting back!

You have reached way down inside yourself, gotten *real* and honest with yourself and decided to get back to where you feel best: back on track! Give yourself a compliment, buy yourself a new outfit, a massage, or something else to reward yourself for your strength, courage, and determination!

REAL WEIGHT

What exactly is your real weight? Everyone is different. Please don't beat yourself up about it like I did for years. It's wasted energy. However, I understand how we can get so caught up in the beauty concept, the "skinny syndrome" and the "land of perfection" expectations. Really, advertising is a major culprit for making us all feel inadequate. I know. I was in the business for seven or eight years. Honestly, there's nothing wrong with striving to improve yourself and a desire to be beautiful... as long as we all realize and acknowledge the very *many* definitions and forms of beauty. What matters is the way *you* think and feel about yourself, not what others think and feel. *Remember: you are loved and accepted exactly as you are, right here, right now. (affirmation by Louise Hay)*

Everyone has their own optimal weight. By optimal, I mean the weight that is healthiest. That is for you to decide. How? Listen to your body.

Again: listen to your body.

Some people say they feel good being overweight. That's fine, but do they know how it feels to be at a healthy weight? Do they remember? Sometimes we get into a comfort zone of being overweight. People adapt to being in a heavier body. Bodies also adapt. Eventually, it gets to the point where we forget how it used to feel when we were at a healthy weight.

On the other hand, some people say they feel good being underweight. Do they really feel good at that weight? Or are they just telling themselves that because they believe thinner is better? Are they struggling to keep their body weight in order to be accepted by others?

Only *you* know how you feel. *You* are the one to decide if you are being honest with yourself.

Yes, there are weight charts that can be used as guidelines. They are just numbers. I believe that feelings are more important than numbers. How you *feel* is much more important. How you feel in your clothes is more important. Many people get caught up in the numbers on the scale. Numbers can be helpful, but they can also torture a person. I stopped weighing myself years ago. My weigh-ins went from being a guideline to a torturous obsession. Be careful with the scale, because your weight is constantly fluctuating. Your body weighs less in the morning than at night. It weighs more when you consume liquids and if you're not eliminating properly. Numbers on the scale can drive you crazy if you are not careful.

After I went too "scale-crazy," I decided I would switch to using my clothes as a guideline. (I don't mean stretch pants or sweatpants. Anything that stretches *that* much is not a guideline; there is too much room for expansion.) Since this change, I have been so much more relaxed about my weight. With clothes as your guideline, you know when to make adjustments. When your "skinny" jeans (or even regular jeans) are getting tight, you know it's time to get your food and exercise in check. Just make sure that your "skinny jeans" are realistic. Someone who has a larger frame is not likely to wear size 2 jeans.

Be honest with yourself. Be kind, but also realistic.

REAL METABOLISM

I'm sure you've heard of people who have a fast or slow metabolism. What does that mean? A scientific explanation would include a total of all chemical reactions that go on inside your body. Metabolism is the rate at which your body burns calories. In fact, 75 percent of the body's energy is used for maintenance. Some maintenance functions are digesting a meal, running a mile, turning the head, and blinking the eyes.

The amount of oxygen your body takes in can affect your metabolism. Our bodies combine oxygen and nutrients to create energy our bodies need for normal bodily functioning. Metabolism is associated with the amount of oxygen your body burns. How do you think people who exercise speed up their metabolism? They're burning calories, fat, and oxygen.

Metabolism occurs in three types: activity, thermic, and basal. Activity metabolism is the amount of energy it takes to perform actively, as in sports, hobbies, housework, and so on. The more active you are, the more you increase your metabolism.

Thermic metabolism is the amount of energy it takes your body to regulate a healthy body temperature. Your body is constantly maintaining its normal temperature of 98.6 °F. This is part of what we call homeostasis (keeping everything in balance within the body). When you are in a hot environment, your body does everything it can to cool down. You sweat when your body gets hot, and this takes energy. Think of it as your body's air conditioner! In a cold environment, your body uses energy to shake and shiver to keep you warm.

Basal metabolism is the caloric energy it takes for your body to function at rest. Believe it or not, you are burning calories all the time. You burn them while you sit, relax, and while you sleep! Even at rest, your body performs many functions. Every time you blink your eyes, take a breath, or feel your heart beat, you are burning calories.

If you have always believed you have a slow metabolism, you are in luck. You *can* change your metabolism. Yes, some people are genetically blessed with a fast metabolism, but you can increase your metabolism by doing certain things.

METABOLISM BOOSTERS (Reproduced As Handout In Appendix)

Exercise

Any form of exercise speeds up the metabolism compared to being sedentary. Take the stairs, do some gardening, walk the dog.

Genetics

Some of us are blessed with a fast metabolism. If you have a fast metabolism, enjoy it. Use it to your advantage, but most of all, appreciate it.

Busyness

The people who cannot sit still increase their metabolism by being busy. All that activity throughout the day adds up. (But please don't take this too much to heart, as we are all too busy with life as it is.)

Sleep

The proper amount of sleep will make your fat burning process more efficient.

Interval Training

Placing more cardiovascular demands on your body speeds up your metabolism.

Strength Training

Placing more strength demands on your body speeds up your metabolism.

A.M. Exercise

Early morning exercise boosts metabolism and benefits you for the rest of the day.

Mental Activity

Mental activity that stimulates *productive* thought helps boost metabolism. The key is being *productive*. Watching TV or playing the same old video games does not qualify.

Small, frequent meals

Digestion helps to speed up metabolism. According to the book "Fit for Life," digestion takes more energy than running, swimming or bike riding. Eating small, frequent meals keeps the fat burning fires going all day. Just make sure you're eating healthy food, or you'll be defeating the whole purpose of speeding up your metabolism.

Eating at the right time of day

Not eating after 8:00 p.m. is important to make the most of digestion and metabolism. There's a saying: *"Eat after eight, gain weight."* If you *really* want to lose weight, don't eat after 5:00 p.m.

Youth

Our metabolism is much faster in our younger years.

Hormones

Balanced hormones can make a huge difference in your metabolism. A simple blood test can help you detect any hormone imbalance so you can correct it and get your metabolism back on track!

Colonics
Colon cleansing improves the efficiency of your digestive tract and elimination system, giving your metabolism a boost.
Pregnancy
Creating a baby is a lot of work! This whole process increases your metabolism.
Breastfeeding
Generating milk for your baby is also extra work for your body and gives your metabolism a boost.

METABOLISM MISTAKES (reproduced as handout in Appendix)
Exercising Too Much
When I studied for my fitness certifications, I learned that excessive exercise makes the body cling to remaining fat. This is a survival mechanism. The body wants to make sure that there is enough fat to keep the body warm and the organs protected.

While teaching fitness classes in Atlanta, I put it to the test. Due to other instructors leaving town for spring break, I taught sixteen fitness classes in one week; sixteen classes in addition to my regular classes. I thought for sure I would lose a few pounds that week. Nope, not one pound. All that extra exercise and not the slightest bit of weight loss.
Inactivity
Living a sedentary lifestyle will give you the metabolism of a snail unless you are genetically blessed.
Sleep deprivation
Lack of sleep will make your fat burning process much slower and less efficient. Sleep is *so* important! Get seven to nine hours, or until you wake up naturally without an alarm clock.
Skipping meals
Skipping meals can lead your body into starvation mode. Since the body does not know when its next meal or calories are coming,

it conserves energy by rationing calorie burn. This slows the body's metabolism.

P.M. Exercise

Exercising in the evening gives your metabolism a boost, but only for a short while. Your metabolism is already slowing down for the day. If that's the best time to exercise for you, by all means, go for it. It will still give your metabolism a boost, just not as much as exercising in the morning.

P.M. Eating

Eating late in the evening is a nightmare—literally. Eating right before bed makes people more likely to have nightmares. Not only does the body lack the time to digest the calories before falling asleep, but it also digests slower due to slower evening metabolism. It's your body's way of winding down for the night. Calories can be stored as fat if not properly digested. Eating during the day is much more efficient than eating in the evening.

Dieting

Extreme changes in the way you eat can mess with your metabolism. A "roller-coaster" way of eating can shift your metabolism in and out of survival mode and causes it to slow down.

Not eating enough calories

Depriving yourself of necessary calories slows metabolism as the body goes into survival mode. Lack of calories tells the body that there may not be enough food in the future. If there is not enough food, the body will go into starvation mode and live off body fat. Once the body is in starvation mode, the metabolism slows down, thus making it more difficult to remove excess body weight.

Alcohol

According to a spa dietician I once worked with, one serving of alcohol slows the metabolism down for a minimum of twenty-four hours after you drink it. One serving means one beer, glass of wine, or one mixed drink. Also, when you eat food along with alcohol, the body processes the alcohol calories first.

Age

Metabolism tends to slow down as we age, but we can get around that by keeping active and following the other metabolism booster tips.

Overeating

Eating too much food at once can cause the body to store excess calories as fat.

Unbalanced hormones

According to a hormone doctor I worked with, once your hormones are balanced, everything else in the body tends to balance out.

THINGS TO KEEP IN MIND ABOUT METABOLISM BEFORE EATING:

Protein

Breaking down protein requires more of your body's energy.

Fiber

Digesting fiber requires more energy, which speeds up metabolism.

Calcium

Calcium helps increase metabolism. Calcium also helps with weight loss.

Spicy Foods

Spicy foods increase metabolism temporarily, although not by much. Don't counteract the benefits by eating something fattening. Keep it healthy.

*Note: *It is not a good idea to consume too much protein or calcium. According to some researchers, consuming too much protein can create an acidic environment within the body. If your body becomes too acidic, calcium can be leached from the bones to help neutralize the acid.*

REAL HORMONES

HORMONE HELL

"Hormone hell" is when your hormones are out of balance and you feel miserable. Symptoms can include any of the following:

*Fatigue/Low energy

*Depression

*Migraines/Headaches

*Weight Gain

*Allergies

*Irregular menstrual cycles

*Bladder issues

*Irritability

*Mood swings

*Decreased sex drive

*Carb Cravings

*Insomnia

*Fibromyalgia

*Memory problems

If you are experiencing such symptoms, you may want to get your hormones checked with a simple blood test. Most insurance companies will pay for the test, but not the hormone balancing program. After you get your results, you can set an appointment with a bioidentical hormone doctor to review your test results and have hormones prescribed if needed. It may take up to three or four months to get your hormones balanced, but once they are, you will feel like a new person—or like the "old you" that used to feel great.

Make sure you get all of your hormones checked with the blood test. (You may want to consider going to a bioidentical hormone doctor before getting the blood test so that the form gets filled out correctly.) All of your hormones may need balancing, or you may just need one simple, over-the-counter, inexpensive hormone called DHEA. The amount of DHEA can affect how well all the other hormones function. For more information, check out the book "Maybe It IS All in Your Head, and You are NOT Crazy."

Some primary care physicians will check a woman's estrogen, progesterone, and thyroid only. It's important to also check your testosterone, cortisol, and DHEA. Your bioidentical hormone doctor may or may not check your cortisol.

HORMONE HEAVEN: BIOIDENTICAL HORMONES

Bioidentical hormones are natural hormones, not synthetic. I used to work with two bioidentical hormone doctors. (See back of book for doctors and office information.) While working there, I learned about hormones and how they can affect your body and life. I observed many women who went from "hormone hell" to "hormone heaven" in just two or three months' time. Before balancing their hormones, many women complained of weight gain even though they were eating healthy and exercising. Some complained of migraines, fatigue, mood swings, memory loss, and decreased sex drive. Men would also complain of weight gain, loss of muscle tone, fatigue and decreased sex drive.

On follow-up visits, most of these people would report major improvements. Some of them appeared to be totally different people with new life in them. They came in feeling great, looking great, and grateful that they had had their hormones balanced. It was very rewarding to see such drastic improvements in these peoples' lives. I was also impressed with how good they felt about themselves. I am not suggesting that this is the ticket for everyone, but I do feel it is at least worth looking into.

REAL SLEEP

Rest? What's that? Not many people know what real rest is. People in this society go a hundred miles an hour, 24/7, day in and day out. When people *do* get some time to themselves, they don't know what to do with it! They are at a loss because they have been going, going, going.

Real rest is about getting seven to nine hours of quality sleep each night. That means no alcohol, cigarettes, or sleeping aids. Real rest is also about getting quality sleep between 10:00 p.m. and 2:00 a.m. During those hours, your body releases healing hormones, creating a deep quality sleep. The catch is, you have to be asleep in order for the healing hormones to release!

If you don't believe me, try it. Go to bed at 10:00 p.m. and sleep for eight hours. Then on another night, go to bed at 2:00 a.m. and sleep for eight hours. Pay attention to how you feel when you get up. Notice the difference in the quality of sleep: how rested or not you feel. Make sure you are fair and treat both nights similarly, meaning no alcohol, cigarettes, or sleep aids on either night. See if you feel a difference.

Real rest is also about having time to yourself. Quality time. Maybe your time is at 5:30 in the morning while everyone else is sleeping. Maybe it's after you get home from work, going into a room and locking the door. Or meditating, taking a warm bath, listening to your favorite relaxing music, or taking a walk out in nature. Whatever it is for you, take the time. You are worth it and you need it. It's healthy to take time to be alone with your thoughts. No interruptions, no other opinions, no phones ringing. Just you and your thoughts.

Taking twenty minutes a day can make a huge difference in how your day goes, how you handle stress, and how you feel about yourself. Know that you are worth it. Where do you squeeze it in? Do you watch TV? Skip it. TV, in my opinion, can be one of the biggest time wasters there is, unless it is an educational program and you are getting something out of it. You have to admit, most programs on television have as much substance as air. In fact, they call TV and radio "air time" in advertising. Most people watch TV out of habit or to zone out. Not much is gained. Most of the information on TV is negative or fear-based. It goes into your brain and stays there, whether you realize it or not. Most people protect themselves from second-hand smoke, so why not protect yourself from brain pollution? Create more time in your day by skipping TV. If you do feel a need to watch TV, watch a program that is educational or entertaining. The problem is that many people become addicted to television, watching any program, just to be watching something. Staying up late to watch TV can also rob you of valuable sleep, making you tired the next day.

Naps are also a luxury if you can squeeze one in. My father used to come home for lunch and lie back in the recliner chair for a fifteen- to twenty-minute nap every work day. He would always go back to work refreshed and ready to go. The key to taking naps is to make sure you get them in before 4:00 p.m.; otherwise you may have a problem getting to sleep later that night. Give your brain and body a break from being bombarded all day long with people, thoughts, advertising, and everything else. *Real rest* is so important. Don't allow yourself to feel guilty for resting. You deserve it. And you'll be so much more productive after a nap. Just make sure you don't nap for more than thirty minutes or you may wake up groggy and more tired than before!

REST/RESTLESS HORMONES

Hormone imbalances can keep us from getting the proper sleep that we all need. A hormone called cortisol helps us cope throughout the day. It peaks in the morning and starts to decline around 3:00 or 4:00 p.m., preparing our bodies to wind down and get ready for sleep. But, because we have stressful days that run past that hour, adrenaline takes over to get us through. The problem is that we are still running on adrenaline when it's time to sleep. So we lie in bed, tossing and turning. We need to slow our bodies down and drain off the adrenaline to get **real rest.**

One way to do this is to do some type of slow repetitive movement for thirty to sixty minutes right before bed each night. Treadmills are great for this. You just walk *very* slowly: 2.5 miles per hour or slower! According to a hormone doctor I worked for, this slow, repetitive movement helps your body lower its adrenaline levels and start making cortisol, helping your body burn three times the fat it would otherwise! Your body has a difficult time burning fat when it's running on adrenaline.

So, shut yourself off from the world for thirty to sixty minutes each night before bed. No phone, no kids, no spouse, no stress. Create a relaxing environment with soft music, or read a book. Whatever you do, don't watch the negative news or a scary movie! That will stress you out and your adrenaline will kick in all over again, putting you right back where you started. If you don't have thirty minutes, try for fifteen. I got this information from Dr. Roby. Try it, it works! You'll sleep deeper and feel so much better when you get up in the morning.

REAL PHYSICAL
HEALING

CHIROPRACTIC

Chiropractors are usually sought out to help alleviate pain. This can be back pain, neck pain, shoulder pain, headaches, numbness, tingling, pinched nerves, or muscle spasms. However, chiropractors may also help align the body. Aligning your skeletal system can make a big difference in improving your health.

I stayed away from chiropractors for years because I could not stand the sound of bones popping. I still don't enjoy the sound, but my eyes were opened when I met a chiropractor who explained the skeletal system to me. Others had laid me down on a table, popping and manipulating my neck, shoulders, and back without a word about what they were doing or why. This brought on not only fear, but confusion.

My most recent holistic chiropractor helped me understand that the spine is more than just a few vertebrae. He informed me about the cerebral spinal fluid and how the health of the spine can affect many other things. He told me how emotion can be stored and blocked within areas of the spine. Once, leaving his office after an adjustment, I found myself crying on the way home— I believe some sort of blockage was removed and the cerebral spinal fluid could now flow the way it was supposed to.

Wellness chiropractors focus on the importance of exercise, nutrition, and overall wellness. Wellness can include emotional health, the use of meditation, and examining the way you deal with stress in your life. These practitioners tend to treat you as a whole being, versus just looking at the symptoms of a problem.

ACUPUNCTURE

Acupuncture also treats the whole body by going to the cause of the problem. Acupuncture is about clearing the meridians within your body. Meridians are invisible channels through which energy circulates throughout the body. If any of your meridians are blocked, you may experience depression or various types of pain. I have heard stories of people claiming that acupuncturists have helped them with allergies, anxiety, asthma, depression, headaches, high blood pressure, low back pain, IBS, arthritis, and weight loss.

An acupuncturist usually uses short, thin needles to open or clear the meridians within the body. The needles are painless. You won't feel anything but a small pin prick at the beginning, if you feel anything at all. In fact, there have been times when I felt as if I'd had a massage after receiving an acupuncture session!

Acupuncture was an effective form of therapy for me when I was experiencing neck and shoulder pain. I went for four or five sessions and was relieved of the pain completely. In fact, the acupuncture session even helped me to release some pent-up emotion. I relaxed and went into a meditative state, and tears trickled down my face as I laid there peacefully. After another relaxing acupuncture session, I left the office and walked to my car. I started to cry uncontrollably. I had no idea where it was coming from, but was aware that the emotion needed to be released. This lasted for about twenty minutes.

I am not saying that you are going to cry if you experience acupuncture. I only experienced that in two of my sessions. All others were peaceful and effective sessions that I appreciated just for the time to lie down and relax!

Benefits of Acupuncture

*Decreased stress	*Calmness
*Increased sense of well-being	*Overcome addictions
*Improved sleep/alleviated insomnia	*Relief of chronic pain
*Relief of headaches/migraines	*Whole body treatment

ESSENTIAL OILS

Natural essential oils can be very healing. Many plants that we take for granted are extremely healing. Their essential oils can help relieve pain, improve your immune system, help you relax and sleep better (or wake you up), or even keep bugs away. These oils are helpful when they complement other forms of holistic therapy.

Essential oils can be inhaled through a vaporizer, massaged into the skin, used in bath water to absorb into the skin externally, or taken internally. Please consult an essential oils practitioner before using oils. Some are for the skin, but some are not. Some are to be taken internally, some are not. And, make sure you purchase oils that are a therapeutic grade. They will give you much better results than the less expensive, average oils.

Peppermint oil is used to relieve headaches, nausea, and to energize. Lemon oil is used for cleaning and for combating the flu, depression, fatigue, and warts. Lavender is great for acne, anxiety, depression, stress, asthma, and for relaxing the mind and body. Basil helps with colds, sinusitis, bronchitis, and is used as an insect repellent. Oils can also be used to balance your chakras. (See Chakra Healing section and Essential Oils chart in Appendix).

BENEFITS OF ESSENTIAL OILS

*Help heal acne
*Calm anger
*Increase confidence
*Alleviate constipation
*Help with concentration
*Decrease stress
*Improve memory
*Improve allergies
*Repel insects
*Improve skin conditions
*Increase relaxation
*Cleanse/anti-septic
*Relieve headaches
And more.

*Help depression
*Calm anxiety
*Help arthritis
*Help relieve fear
*Reduce insecurities
*Promote energy
*Build immune system
*Reduce pain
*Soothe insect bites
*Improve sleep
*Balance emotions
*Help cramps
*Improve memory

REAL WATER/AIR

Real water means purified water; the purer the water, the purer your body. The type of water you consume is very important. Your body is 70 percent water. You need water to survive. Water hydrates you, cleanses you, and helps your body to function properly.

Hydration is so important. Dehydration can lead to headaches, fatigue, muscle tightness, joint discomfort, toxemia, dry skin, and constipation. Think back to that hangover you once had. Did you wake up with a headache? The alcohol you drank the night before dehydrated you overnight. The same thing happens when you don't drink enough water daily. Keeping your body hydrated will help keep you energized. Dehydration can fatigue you, so if you are feeling tired, drink water.

Water also helps keep your muscles flexible and joints running smoothly. Not enough water in the muscles and joints creates inflexibility and stiffness. According to the book, "Living without Pain, by Harvey Diamond, toxins also collect in the joints. Water is a big help in flushing out the toxins within your body.

Water also helps with weight loss. Whoa! That's usually enough of a reason right there for most people to drink water. Excess weight is additional fat cells if overfed before birth, during infancy or adolescent growth phase. During other times of our lives, it can also be an expansion of fat cells that we already have,   Some researchers believe that excess weight is an accumulation of toxins within the fat tissue. Drinking enough water is the best way to flush your body out. Cleanse it.

Water helps keep your skin moist. It also helps keep your bowels moving. Anytime you are constipated, drink water. Water helps the colon absorb nutrients and eliminate toxic waste. The more toxic waste you eliminate, the healthier you'll be. If your colon becomes dehydrated because your body is dehydrated, then that toxic waste does not get eliminated. If it does not get eliminated, it gets backed up. If it gets backed up...you become more toxic! Also, the more waste you release, the less you'll weigh!

Tap water is not the best choice, although it is much better in some cities than others. Look up your city tap water on the Internet and see where it stands in water purity. There is a debate about the lack of fluoride in purified water. Some say fluoride is harmful to your body, others say a lack of fluoride can promote tooth decay. Something to think about. Research the subject and you decide. I personally drink both. *Balance!*

Some people say that distilled water is the purest. However, distilled water is also known to leach minerals out of your body, according to the book "Staying Healthy with Nutrition." The minerals have been "purified" out of distilled water. Our bodies need minerals, just as it needs vitamins. The challenge is to get pure water with no harmful bacteria yet which retains the helpful minerals.

There are many good purification products to choose from. Some are more expensive than others, depending on the quality of water you want. Just remember that water is 70 percent of what you are made of. Do you want to be 70 percent bacteria-ridden? 70 percent chlorine-ridden? 70 percent fluoride-free? 70 percent mineral-free? Or 70 percent pure?

I have been using the Multi-Pure system for many years. It is a carbon filter purifier. The filter needs to be replaced every year or sooner, depending on the number of people in your household and the amount of water that is filtered. You may also want to consider getting a chlorine filter for your shower head. Those also need a filter replacement every year, or sooner if there are more than two people in your household. These filters can help protect your skin from dryness and chemicals being absorbed into your body. Many people are not aware that our skin is the largest organ of our body. Keep in mind that chemicals from many different sources that you put on your skin can be absorbed through your pores.

Whatever the case, do your body a favor and make sure it receives enough water—purified water, if possible. Just know that there are pros and cons to all kinds.

The chlorine in swimming pools can be absorbed into your body as can germs and bacteria. If you must use a pool, do what you can to rinse your body off after swimming. That way, chlorine and bacteria are not sitting on your skin any longer than necessary. I sure took the fun out of the summer activity of swimming, didn't I? Sorry! I just want to inform you of what your body puts up with there. I personally love going to the pool, but I rarely go into the water. I use the environment to relax, read, and get my vitamin D. Only when it is super hot will I get in to cool off. When it is that hot, more often I skip the pool and stay inside. There are swimming pools now that are filled with salt water instead of using chlorine. Check them out and see which is best for you.

REAL AIR
AIR PURIFIERS

Air? Gotta have it! The question is, what type of air are you breathing? Clean? Dirty? Chemical-ridden? Pollution-filled? First-hand smoke? Second-hand smoke? Pollen- or mold-ridden air? Or fresh mountain air?

If you are not breathing fresh, clean mountain air, you may want to consider using an air filter at home. Every breath you take can make a big difference in the health of your body. We all know that breathing smoke is not healthy. Avoid smoke or polluted air when you can.

If you are a smoker or are exposed to polluted or chemical-ridden air, try using a Rife machine. The Rife machine booklet has a frequency for lungs, allergies and emphysema. After doing a lung session on the Rife machine I felt my lungs expand and able to breathe so much better the next day. I do it at night while I am sleeping.

Note: *If you live in the country, breathe in. Country air is so much better for your health. Appreciate it.*

REAL SUNSHINE HEALTH

HEALING EFFECTS OF THE SUN

The sun is very healing to the body, mind and spirit. We have been brainwashed into believing the sun is harmful and not to be out in it unless you are covered in SPF 90 sunscreen! Have you noticed that the sunscreen SPFs are getting higher and higher? At the same time, skin cancer is on the rise. Countries that have the highest use of sunscreen have the highest rates of skin cancer. Richard Hobday, author of *The Healing Sun*, states that using a sunscreen which blocks out UVB radiation to prevent burning might also stop the synthesis of vitamin D, a reduction of cholesterol levels and lowering of blood pressure. I know that everyone tells us that we should fear the sun. I disagree. I know what feels good to me and my body and I believe that the sun is healing. Now, if you abuse the power of the sun, yes, it can be harmful. Many things can be harmful if abused. Too much or too little of a lot of things is not good. Fifteen to twenty minutes of morning or late afternoon sunshine is enough for your body's vitamin D requirement.

Different parts of the country and the world experience different levels of sun intensity. There is also the ozone factor. The ozone layer is a layer in the earth's atmosphere that contains high levels of ozone.

evels can cause harmful effects on the respiratory systems of animals and can burn sensitive plants.

Let's just think about this....Really...What did the cavemen do when they were alive? Do you think they put on sunscreen before they stepped outside their caves? Don't think so...They obviously survived without sunscreen. Some people believe that the diet of the caveman included many dark leafy greens which contain chlorophyll. Chlorophyll helps protect the skin from getting sunburned.

When I was a 100% raw foodist, my skin never burned while out in the sun. The raw foodists' theory was that the chlorophyll in the dark leafy greens acted as a natural sunscreen.

Have you ever noticed how good it feels to see the sun after two to three days of rain and overcast weather? The sun feels so good on your face that first spring day after three or four months of the winter cold. The sun tends to lift our spirits and rejuvenate us. The sun feels good to people and to animals. Dogs sunbathe in the yard. Cats sunbathe by the window. Snakes sunbathe in the grass or on rocks. And turtles sunbathe on logs. The sun can't be all bad if everyone's basking in it!

The sun also provides vitamin D in its the best form. I have been a sun goddess for years. And I don't wear sunscreen, except for on my nose and lips. Now, I will tell you that I have abused the sun in the past. Years ago, when sunbathing, it felt so good that I overdid it, too many times. I have gotten sunburn, freckles and wrinkles from it. But that is my fault, not the sun's. I am responsible for how large a sunshine dose I give myself. I should know when enough is enough. It is my responsibility to remove myself from the sun or cover up.

You don't need a large dose of the sun, in fact, it's best to get it in small doses. Fifteen to twenty minutes a day on your hands and/or face is sufficient. The best time to get sunshine therapy is within the first four hours of sunrise and within the last four hours prior to sunset. The most beneficial time of year to get sunshine is spring and early summer. However, it is important to receive sunshine all year round. That may be difficult in the northern states, but it is possible.

The good thing about Vitamin D is that the body is able to store it—but please make sure you get your daily dose. A deficiency of vitamin D can create rickets, a softening of the bones, so get outside, even if it's only for a few minutes. According to the book, "The Healing Sun," sunshine can help lower cholesterol and blood pressure as well as help heal some forms of acne and eczema. Other disorders like breast cancer, heart disease, multiple sclerosis and osteoporosis can be helped by sunlight.

Sunlight also enters the body through your eyes. Being out in the sun without glasses, sunglasses and/or contacts helps to stimulate the pineal gland. (The pineal gland, having many functions, acts as the light meter of the body and also sends out hormonal messages.) According to the book, *Light: Medicine of the Future*, receiving sunlight through your eyes is the best way to absorb the sunlight. It helps improve eyesight and the immune system.

Make an effort to get outside. Get your vitamin D while walking the dog, gardening, doing lawn work, playing Frisbee, or just sunbathing. Not only is it relaxing, but it's good for you!

REAL NATURE

Nature is extremely healing and helps to reduce stress. *Real nature* can be anything from walking on a trail or driving to your favorite scenic spot to relax next to a waterfall. This is one of the activities that a lot of people neglect to do. Nature is very often taken for granted.

HIKING

I've been a nature lover for years and have experienced a lot of nature over twelve years of hiking. I always come back more relaxed and at peace. While out hiking, I have come up with creative ideas, solutions to problems, cried my eyes out, or felt sheer joy from the experience of being in nature. My hikes usually range from sixty to ninety minutes. Although that amount of time spent in nature is a luxury for your soul, even twenty minutes can be very beneficial. You don't have to hike. You can just sit and relax, soaking up the beauty. You'll become a different person. Not only is it time for yourself, it is healing time. Healing energy from the trees and plants help to rejuvenate your mind, body, and soul. I recommend getting out in nature at least once a week—every day if possible. Try it for a month and see the benefits that come from it.

ANIMAL SIGHTINGS AND SYMBOLISM

Next time you are out in nature, look closely at all that surrounds you. Pay attention to the trees, rocks, insects and animals. You may just get an education as well as a break from the craziness of life!

According to the book "Animals Speak," by Ted Andrews, animals can often guide us, send us messages, or warn us about various events that are going on in our lives. The symbolism they hold can help us to identify with what is going on in our lives.

ANIMAL SYMBOLISM (reproduced as a handout in Appendix)

Bear	Trust your inner voice
Bees	Fertility, sexuality, productivity, accomplishing the impossible, enjoying the sweetness of life
Butterfly	Transformation, dancing, joy, lightheartedness, new birth
Blackbird	Promise, protect what you own
Bluebird	Happiness
Canary	Voice, trust your voice
Cardinal	Monogamy, courtship, relationships, feminine side, the number 12, attend to health, self-importance
Cat	Independence, mystery
Cougar	Leadership, strength, staying on track with goals, self-empowerment
Coyote	Trickery, wisdom, trust the plan
Cricket	Good luck, finding light, protection of home, beliefs, trust intuition
Crow	Magical help with problems
Deer	Power of gentleness, innocence, new adventures
Dragonfly	Efforts are coming to fruition, time to shine
Dog	Faithfulness, loyalty, protection of self and surroundings
Dove	Peace, new opportunities
Duck	Emotions to be soothed
Eagle	Vision, spirit, spiritual

Fox	Beware of camouflaged surroundings, do not reveal your plan, shifting situations, magic
Frog	Transformation, emotions, water
Gecko	Take action
Hawk	Guiding vision, observe, opportunities, surrounding guardianship
Horse	Freedom, strength, beauty, grace, power, new journeys ahead
Humming-bird	Joy
Ladybug	Wish fulfilled
Lion	Strength of will
Lizard	Dreams, intuition, pay attention to dreams and psychic feelings
Mouse	Focus on details
Owl	Wisdom, moon, hear what is hidden, spirits
Praying Mantis	Stillness, be patient for success
Rabbit	Overcoming fear, wait for answers
Raccoon	Disguise, masking is happening
Roadrunner	Speed, to think quickly
Scorpion	transformation, sexual needs, passion
Snake	Rebirth, transformation, healing, protector, shed the old skin
Spider	Weaving fate, trust feeling, not what you see
Squirrel	Gather, prepare, busyness, conserve, work and play
Tiger	Power, assert power
Toad	Emotional cleansing, transformation, inner strength, good luck, money
Turtle	Promise, take your time
Wasp	Protection around you
Wolf	Spirit guide, loyalty, intuition, learning, inner strength, protected, trust in self

To find symbolism of animals not listed, look up the animal you'd like to know about on Google, using its name and the phrase "animal symbolism."

Example: alligator animal symbolism

SAVE THE EARTH

Earth: the word means different things to different people.

Is it just dirt?

Or is it dirt that covers the ground and helps the trees to grow and that provide oxygen for us to breathe, the trees that create a home for the chirping birds and the frisky squirrels. This is the dirt that grows fruits and vegetables so we can have them on our dinner tables to nourish our healthy bodies.

This is also the same dirt that creates the beautiful wildflowers that cover the fields—the flowers that we enjoy smelling and looking at, the flowers that we buy for our loved ones.

Earth is "dirt," yes, but, it is so much more. It is our planet. It's our home. Why go out of your way to save the earth? Because, it's the only one we've got, just as we only have one body. We need to take care of it and respect it.

That's what *Earth Day* is about. It is a day to respect the earth, a day to remind us all to continue caring for our precious planet. It's a day to check in with ourselves and ask if we are doing all we can to save it.

Are you making a negative impact on the earth or a positive one? There are ways to calculate your carbon footprint. Go online. It takes three minutes. What can you do to save the earth? Recycle, plant a tree, pick up litter. Everyone can do something to save the earth.

Feel good about yourself and where you live…Save the earth!

HEALING STONES/CRYSTALS

Stones give off healing energies, help absorb negative energies and also deflect negative energies. Healing stones may also provide health, wealth, growth and protection. I became interested in healing stones and crystals when going through chakra healing therapy. If you have certain blockages on your heart or any of your chakras (see Energy Healing), try a healing stone. Healing stones can help heal a broken heart, pain from loss, rid you of fear and improve many physical ailments.

I am not an expert in the field, but believe in the healing energy of stones and wear them every day. They come in bracelets, anklets, pendants, charms, earrings and as loose stones. I wear them around my neck, wrists, ankles, and ears. Some loose stones are carried in my purse. It's interesting to research all the different stones, what they symbolize and how they heal. I recommend researching any stones that you are drawn to. The stones you are drawn to are usually the ones you need most.

Most healing stones need to be cleansed through the sun, the moon (full moon), dry sea salt, or with cool water. Light from the moon cleanses the negative energy that some stones tend to absorb or pick up from other people. Research your stones before cleansing them, because some will fade from the sun, so you can put those out under a full moon overnight. (See Healing Stones chart in Appendix)

* * *

SECTION III:

REAL WELLNESS

EMOTIONAL HEALTH &
HEALING
POSITIVE ATTITUDE &
ENVIRONMENT

REAL RELATIONSHIPS

Everyone is involved in a relationship at some point in life. The question is, what kind of relationship is it? Are you in a healthy relationship or an unhealthy, dysfunctional relationship? People say that relationships are a lot of work. How much work should they be? I look at it this way: if you experience more drama than joy in your relationship, then it is going to take a lot of work. It may take so much work that it drains and exhausts you to the point of wanting to give up or just be single. Yes, I do believe that relationships take work, but you shouldn't have to be arguing every weekend or draining all of your energy just to keep it going.

Look at what percentage of your relationship is relaxing, fun and joyful, and what percent of it is work, drama, and exhaustion. If you are exhausted 70 to 80 percent of the time on a regular basis, then you may be incompatible with someone. I have had different relationships—some easy and flowing and some quite challenging. There are pros and cons to either situation. Some flowing relationships may be easy but boring. On the other hand, the passionate relationships can be drama-filled and exhausting.

We can ask ourselves which extreme we want to live with, or we can work on ourselves and experience a relationship that is healthy and functional, yet still filled with passion and joy. The "work," in my opinion, is how much you work on yourself. Many people go through one long-term relationship, or many short-term relationships, learning a different lesson from each relationship. Others repeat the same pattern over and over again, wondering what happened. They wonder why they keep ending up with the same problems over and over again with the same person or many different people.

When a relationship ends, it may mean that it's served its purpose, or it may mean there was work that needed to be done. If you are repeating a cycle in your relationships (which many people do), then it's likely that you'll continue to repeat it, even if you're with a different person.

We can move beyond our destructive cycles by taking a look at ourselves. Sorry to say this, but it's not always the other person's fault the way most of us would like to think. There are two sides to every story. As I said earlier in this book, you are not always right.

I once heard a question in one of the self-growth trainings that I attended in Dallas: "Do you want to be right, or do you want to be happy?" That is a question to ponder. What is more important to you? Being right or being happy? Now, I am not saying that you should allow the other person to be right all the time and walk all over you in order to keep the peace. That does not lead to true happiness.

True happiness (or what I like to call joy), is *being* at peace and knowing that we are not all perfect. None of us are. We all make mistakes, we all have issues and we all have patterns that are set early in childhood. I may sound like Freud here, but we tend to learn our patterns from our parents (or guardians) in childhood.

One of our challenges in life is to figure out who we are, why we do certain things, and how to combat the negative and replace it with the positive. Some situations take a lot of therapy, some take a lot of understanding, and some take major wake-up calls.

Therapy, understanding, and wake-up calls can help us to become aware of what we are doing in relationships. We can be aware of our own behavior and our partner's, or we can go through life in total ignorance, not paying attention to anything about ourselves or anyone.

Real relationships, I believe, are relationships that lift you up and help you grow. *Real relationships* are the ones where both parties are aware of their own behavior and consciously correct it. If we continue to avoid who we are and what we do to ourselves and others, then we are pretty much destined to take the long route to joy and happiness.

Years ago, I read a book called *A Return to Love: Reflections on the Principles of A Course in Miracles* by Marianne Williamson. Although it was many, many years ago, I do remember one main message from the book. Once you stop finding fault and blaming the other person and take a good look at yourself, that's when you get that wake-up call. When you take action and work to make yourself a better person, that's when you start attracting different types of people. You start progressing and evolving in relationships. Now, I'm not saying that your work is done after that—but it definitely lifts you to a higher level.

Once you have reached that higher level, you tend to vibrate at a different frequency. The people that were once attracted to you are now attracted to the people you used to be like. After you've worked on yourself, looked at your own behavior, and have come to understand why you do what you do, more evolved people will be attracted to you. The "old" you is gone, and the new you is emerging. You are still learning, but without the same old patterns that you once repeated.

EGO LOVE VS. REAL LOVE

There are all different kinds and levels of love. Without going into all of them, I would like to discuss two forms of love: *ego-based* love and *Real Love.* Ego-based love comes from the ego or the mind. Real love comes from the heart and soul.

Ego-based love originates from what we think love is or "should" be. The ego mind takes us to a place of expectations, negativity, and "shoulds." When we are experiencing ego-based love, we tend to expect many things from others. We think too much and don't *feel* enough. Ego love is love that we think we need *from another*. Ego love comes from others instead of from within ourselves. Ego love finds fault in others when they do not meet our expectations. Ego love leaves us feeling unfulfilled and lacking. Ego love is never enough to satisfy us. It is insatiable. It keeps us constantly trying to please, only to find that whatever we give is not enough.

The ego is all in our mind and keeps us unhappy, frustrated, and feeling unloved. Our egos tend to overthink everything that others are doing or not doing. The ego tends to keep us miserable in a world where enough is never enough. The ego is never satisfied. It is pleased only temporarily, only to find a feeling of emptiness again. The ego makes us think we have to be "right." It keeps us arguing because it is never satisfied with what it receives. No matter how hard another tries to love us or please us, the ego finds something wrong with the relationship or situation.

Ego love is about jealousy, pride, negativity, and control. The ego likes to have the upper hand and does not want to admit its own wrongdoing. Ego love does not want to be vulnerable because the ego feels that showing vulnerability is weakness. The ego has a need to be strong all the time and has a difficult time apologizing. Overall, ego love is about being in the head, not the heart. It doesn't care if it is fair, patient, or understanding. Ego love wants what it wants, when it wants it. The ego is not *real*.

Real love is very different from ego love. *Real love* is about being accepting, healthy, and understanding. *Real love* is fair, trusting, and vulnerable. *Real love* functions without having to be in control. It is about freedom: freedom for both parties to be who they truly are. *Real love* is about trust and honesty. *Real love* operates from the heart and soul. *Real love* is about authentic apologies and forgiveness. *Real love* wants the best for everyone's highest good.

CHARACTERISTICS OF EGO-BASED LOVE VS. REAL LOVE:

Ego-based Love	Real Love
*Jealous	*Self-confident
*Distrusting	*Trusting
*Unhealthy	*Healthy
*Heavy	*Light
*Controlling	*Freeing
*Conditional	*Unconditional
*Listening (but not hearing)	*Hearing
*Disrespectful	*Respectful
*Full of confusion	*Clear
*Chaotic	*Peaceful
*Non-communicative	*Communicative
*Sorrowful	*Joyful
*Head-based	*Heart-based
*Expects	*Accepts
*Dysfunctional	*Functional
*Toxic	*Cleansed
*Rollercoaster-like	*Stable
*Ungrateful	*Grateful
*Impatient	*Patient
*Hard	*Soft
*Cold	*Warm
*Cruel	*Kind
*Unsatisfied	*Satiated
*Needy	*Fulfilled
*Desperate	*Assured

*Intolerable	*Tolerable
*Cowardly	*Courageous
*Sedentary	*Motivated
*Sad	*Cheerful
*Depressing	*Uplifting
*Unsupportive	*Supportive
*Draining	*Filling
*Exhausting	*Energizing
*Aimless	*Directed
*Sabotaging	*Healing
*Flighty	*Grounding
*Unbalanced	*Balanced
*Stagnating	*Growing
*Destructive	*Creative
*Apathetic	*Empathetic
*Insensitive	*Sensitive
*Without compassion	*Compassionate
*Disharmonious	*Harmonious
*Unfaithful	*Faithful
*Low in self-esteem	*High in self-worth
*Weakening	*Strengthening
*Discouraging	*Encouraging
*Low in self-love	*High in self-love
*Unequal	*Equal
*Unaligned	*Aligned
*Withholding	*Expressive
*Argumentative	*Discussion-oriented
*Taking	*Giving
*Unaffectionate	*Affectionate
*Removed	*Close
*Stressed	*Carefree

*Unhappy	*Happy
*Pessimistic	*Optimistic
*Stormy	*Calm
*Weak	*Strong and lasting
*Uptight	*Relaxed
*Emotionally unavailable	*Emotionally available
*Spiritually unavailable	*Spiritually available
*Physically unavailable	*Physically available
*Dirty fighting	*Fighting fair
*Immature	*Mature
*Partial	*Whole
*Physical	*Spiritual
*Sex	*Lovemaking
*Being something we are not	*Being what we truly are
*Dishonest	*Honest
*Closed	*Open
*Negative	*Positive
*Empty	*Full
*Act out of obligation	*Act out of desire
*About " being right"	*About being happy and fair
*One-sided	*Two-sided
*Based on thought	*Based on feeling
*Unconscious	*Conscious
*Unaware	*Aware
*Ego-based	*Soul-based
*Based on fear	*Based on Love

EGO LOVE (TOXIC RELATIONSHIPS)

We are all programmed from childhood to repeat patterns that we learned from our parents. Haven't you wondered why you keep attracting men like your father? Or women like your mother? That's great if your mother or father was perfect. But really, none of us are perfect, not even our parents. Just know that they did the best they could, based on their own upbringing and knowledge. Like you, they learned from their parents and had many things to attend to while raising you. People can only do so much. If they were not given the tools to be perfect parents, then they most likely made some mistakes. Do your best to forgive them, but be aware of the things that need correcting.

Toxic relationships are dysfunctional and unhealthy. They repeat the same old pattern over and over again. They can be very frustrating, draining, and exhausting. You know what I am talking about: the constant fights, the jealousy, the insecurities, and the nonstop draining discussions about "the relationship." When you continue to discuss the same issues over and over again with no positive results, you are wasting time, energy, and emotion. Usually these types of arguments are based on ego, not love. The ego has to be right, while *Real Love seeks to communicate and understand.*

The reason we repeat patterns is because we are functioning out of reactions instead of being aware.

When you are not aware, you react. You are in your head, not your heart, and this leads the relationship into toxicity. When your relationship is toxic, you tend to feel confused about why it doesn't seem to progress.

These relationships can be very detrimental until you become aware. When you do, you see yourself, your partner, and the relationship as if you were standing outside of the situation—something like watching a movie. You tend to pick up clues to various behaviors and realize things about yourself and your partner. Becoming aware that you're in a toxic relationship is the first step toward healing and correcting dysfunctional behaviors. Until you can see yourself and what you are doing, you cannot change your behavior.

When you are in your heart, you are calm, nonreactive, and hearing your partner (and yourself). You are an attentive listener and aware of what is going on in the conversation. You can catch yourself going from your heart to your head. When this happens, you must stop the thought, word, or reaction in the moment and choose a different thought, word, or action. Everything starts with thought. In fact, *the only thing we are ever dealing with is a thought. And a thought can be changed. (Louise Hay)*

Being aware in a relationship helps you to make healthier choices. If you can remain conscious during dysfunctional behavior, you can change it in the moment. Remaining conscious like this can be challenging, but it is possible. It takes a lot of practice to stay aware of what is going on, what you are doing, and what your partner is doing, especially in a heated moment. Once you are able to observe the relationship through new eyes, you can work on changes.

I know. I have been in toxic relationships that were full of arguments, heaviness, and frustration. I was attracted to men who were controlling, domineering, negative, critical, and sometimes alcoholic. A day came when I realized that I kept having unfulfilling relationships and decided to make a change. I started out by reading books. In the past, I had read books on relationships but never really did the exercises in them. I felt that it wasn't necessary, or that it just took too much time. Little did I know that actually doing the exercises would help me to release my feelings and see that I truly was repeating patterns.

One exercise was to list the significant men in my past and their negative qualities. Once I completed it, I sat back and saw, in writing, how all the men I had dated were very similar. This was a huge eye-opener for me.

I considered going to a counselor, yet hesitated for some time because I had a degree in psychology. I felt that I should have known how to have a healthy relationship. But the thought that maybe I was too close to the situation made me consider that an outsider might be able to see behaviors that I was not seeing. *It's not always an easy thing, to see ourselves.*

That's when I decided to seek some form of counseling. Not because I was crazy, but because I did not want to continue participating in relationships that were unfulfilling. I was tired of the same old behaviors and disappointing results. I had reached a point in my life where I felt I deserved to have a healthy, loving, fulfilling relationship.

BEING A VICTIM

Being a victim is about "poor me." The "poor me" syndrome keeps you stuck. It immobilizes you. I ran across this saying a couple of years ago: *"You cannot be powerful if you are pitiful."* Makes you think, doesn't it? Being a victim can be very comfortable for a while. I'm sure we've all had our moments when we were victims. Some of us have had more than moments: we've had days, weeks, or years as victims.

I am not saying that you should not be upset or feel emotion when something terrible happens to you. What I *am* saying is that staying a victim can be detrimental to your health, your growth, and your soul.

One advantage of being a victim is that you get to be lazy. It keeps you stuck, going nowhere. It helps you justify the act of doing nothing about your situation. Being a victim gives you an excuse to sit back and feel sorry for yourself.

Another advantage is that you get *so* much sympathy from others. There are a lot of sympathetic people out there. If one doesn't feel sorry for you, then next one will. If someone close to you gets fed up with your pity party, they may choose to step away. That's ok, because we tend to gravitate toward those who support our victimization.

There are a lot of horrible things that happen in the world. Feeling emotion about them is normal. We're human. Releasing that emotion (in a healthy way) is great. But staying stuck in "poor me" gets old.

It gets so old, so fast, that you'll notice even the sympathizers step away after a while, because it is so draining. But full-time victims always seem to smell out new sympathizers, until they wear them out, also.

I know; I had to let a friend of mine go a few years back. This friend was draining my energy so badly that it was starting to affect my health. I had no energy for my daughter, who needed me, or for myself. I finally reached a point where I became aware of what I was doing, and how it was affecting my life and my daughter's life. I decided to take action.

No matter how I attempted to help this friend, it was never enough. There was guilt on my part, but I soon realized that I needed to save myself or I would be taken down. It was as if I were trying to save someone from drowning, but the person I was trying to save was splashing about and panicking so much that she was pulling me down with her. I was starting to drown. I was exhausted, drained, depressed, and so tired. The life had been sucked out of me. That's when I said "Enough" and let her go.

I'm sure she found someone new: someone who was rested and refreshed, ready to take on her victimization. But I was done. The final straw was when she told me that I was never there for her. That was it! Not only had I given up my time, energy and emotion for this woman, but I was now not even worth an acknowledgment. I wasn't expecting a thank you, but refusing to acknowledge that I had been there for her? Done.

It felt strange to let a friend go like that, but I realized that this was not the first time it had happened and that it had been a very one–sided relationship. I gave and she took, over and over and over again until she wore me out. Being a single mom, my time and energy was precious. My daughter and I both deserved to have it.

Little did I know how much lighter my life would become after I let my friend go. It was as if someone had lifted a hundred pounds off my shoulders. It's been years, and I have no regrets about what I did. In fact, looking back I realize that what I did was honor myself. It was also a way of showing myself self-love.

REAL SELF-LOVE/ EMPOWERMENT

Self-love is about fulfilling your needs, whether they be physical, mental, emotional, or spiritual. We all have needs and we all deserve to have them met. The kicker is to realize that we are responsible for realizing what our needs are. Nobody else can tell us, and we are all different. When one person may need a hug, another person may need food in the stomach. We are the ones who know ourselves best. We are responsible for figuring out what our needs are, and then to communicate those needs to others so that they can be met. If someone else cannot help you with a particular need, you are responsible for getting it met, or finding someone who *can* help you.

Sometimes we expect others to know what our needs are. It's as if we expect them to read our minds. No one can do that. If we are not aware of what our needs are and don't communicate them clearly, we become needy. When we constantly rely on others to figure out our needs, we become needy, dependent, and miserable.

Being needy or dependent is usually not very becoming. Not only that, but when we are needy or dependent, we give up control of our lives. We give our power to others. If you like being powerless, that's your choice. If you choose to own your power, then take it back. Take control of your life.

Self-love is about figuring out what your needs are, communicating them, and getting them met. Self-love is about owning your power, taking control of your life, and living it in a way that honors who you are.

HONORING YOURSELF

Honoring yourself is being true to yourself. Being true to yourself is listening to your inner voice, trusting it, and acting on it. Listening is easy because the voice never goes away. Trusting it, however, can be a challenge. Trust yourself. If you have a problem trusting other people, you may want to take a look at yourself. Ask yourself if you trust yourself. Trusting yourself is about doing what you need to do for you to be "right" with yourself and honor your own feelings. If you feel upset about something that someone said or did, maybe you need to speak up about it. If someone has degraded you or hurt you, honoring yourself would be to correct the situation. If you are feeling guilty because you hurt someone, correct it. Or, as Bernie from Millennium 3 Education would say, "Clean it up."

Confronting the person or the situation can be uncomfortable, but so can living with guilt, resentment, or anger. Setting it right within you may not involve confronting someone. It may involve writing a letter or journaling—whatever it is you need to do to be true to yourself and your feelings, do it.

I am not talking about getting revenge or "getting back at" someone for what they did to you. That would be adding more negativity to the situation. I am talking about what you can do to make peace with yourself and/or another person in a healthy way, so you can let it go. Letting it go sets you free. Letting it go brings peace.

Honoring yourself may be something as simple as taking yourself out dancing because you deserve to smile, laugh, hear music, and enjoy yourself. It could be getting some exercise because your body needs it and misses it. Honoring yourself could be stepping away from a toxic relationship. Maybe your soul has been telling you this for some time now and you are now hearing it, trusting it, and acting on it.Honoring yourself may be forgiving someone who hurt you. Maybe you have been punishing them repeatedly for the same mistake. Maybe honoring yourself is to give them peace and set them free with your *authentic* forgiveness.

Honoring yourself may mean forgiving yourself. We tend to forgive others for wrongdoing, but why is it so hard to forgive ourselves? Do we not honor or value ourselves? Forgiving yourself is definitely a big way to honor yourself. It helps you to forgive others. You are just as important as anyone else. No one is more important than you. No one's feelings are more important than yours.

Honor yourself. Value yourself. Be true to yourself. Love yourself. Forgive yourself. Be at peace with yourself.

Be yourself. Be *Real!*

VALUING YOURSELF: BOUNDARIES

Self-worth is about standing up for yourself, speaking your mind, honoring your feelings, speaking your truth, and setting boundaries.

There is a saying: *"We teach people how to treat us."* That's what setting boundaries does. If we allow people to walk all over us we are saying, "You can treat me badly. I don't mind." If we allow people to lie, cheat, hurt, control, or manipulate us, we send a message to them that says, "It's okay to treat me badly." Allowing people to say or do negative things to us tells them that we do not value or respect ourselves.

We can place blame on the person who is hurting us, but doing so makes us a victim and leaves us powerless. When we stand up for ourselves, set boundaries, and enforce them, we tell people that we value ourselves and will not tolerate that type of behavior or treatment. It sends a message that we are important and that we respect ourselves; that their negative or hurtful behavior is unacceptable.

Valuing yourself empowers you and puts you in control of your life. I know, because I allowed a past boyfriend to treat me negatively. This treatment included verbal and emotional abuse. When I stood up for myself, he would use guilt to control and manipulate me. The guilt was *my* issue. I allowed myself to feel guilty again and again. I thought that I liked, loved, and valued myself, but came to realize that I was not valuing myself enough. I had stood up for myself verbally, but not backed it up with action. Backing it up with action includes setting boundaries and enforcing them.

Heck, I didn't even know what my boundaries were for a long time. How then, could I set them and enforce them? I read a book on boundaries that enlightened me…I mean, *really* enlightened me.

So I started setting boundaries, yet he kept crossing them. I let this boyfriend know that crossing my boundaries was disrespectful and unacceptable. When he continued, I terminated the relationship. *(You cannot change other people's behavior, but you CAN change your own behavior.)* Once I ended the relationship, I felt incredible. I felt light, happy, and free…so free. I started to value myself at work and in other relationships. My world started to open up. Everything that had felt negative became positive. Life had taken on new meaning, all because I learned to value myself.

Do yourself and your life a favor. Teach others how to treat you: value yourself. Set boundaries. Enforce them. You will feel your value go up!

REAL LOVE

Real Love starts with you. When you *truly* love yourself, you'll be ready to be in a true love relationship. Loving yourself is key, though getting there can be a challenge. Loving yourself is about treating yourself like you would your best friend. It is about taking good care of your body, mind and spirit. This can include stimulating your mind with positive thoughts, exercising your body, feeding it healthy, nourishing foods, and listening to your soul. Exercising your mind, then giving it a rest… exercising your body, then giving it a rest…listening, trusting, and acting on your soul.

Acting on your soul can be doing whatever your soul tells you that you need to do to be on the right path or to be at peace. Acting on your soul can also be giving yourself a break, a rest, some relaxation…a Soul Activity. That's what I call an activity that feeds your soul. (See Soul Activities section)

Real love is also about being comfortable in your own skin. Being able to enjoy your own company is a sign that someone else will also enjoy it. Spending time with others is healthy, but so is spending time with yourself.

Real love in a relationship is loving, giving, receiving, understanding, listening, being true to yourself and your partner, honoring your feelings and your partner's. *Real love* lifts you up, supports you, encourages you and picks you up when you fall.

Real love does not judge, criticize, or degrade you. When your soul is speaking to you, you know; it's that deeply honest inner voice that never seems to go away. Listen. Most of the time, listening to your inner voice is easy; the challenge is to trust it and act on it.

Real love is about commitment, trust, communication, honesty, and respect. You must have all of these things within yourself in order to give them to your partner. This means you must be committed to yourself, communicate your true feelings, be honest with yourself, and respect yourself. Once you develop these qualities within yourself, you may receive and enjoy the same qualities from someone else.

If you are not there yet, remember that we are all growing, every day. Don't be hard on yourself, but do be open to looking at yourself and what you can enhance inside. The love within you is already there. There may be a need to heal all of the self-doubt, insecurities, and/or emotional wounds. Once these wounds have been healed, you'll be on your way to *real love*. (For ways to heal emotional wounds, see the Therapy and Mirror Work section.)

REAL CHOICES

LIFE CHOICES

Every moment of our lives, we are making choices. You choose whether you want to eat, not eat, exercise, not exercise, smile, cry, laugh, dance, think negatively, or think positively. We choose how we react to things. We choose to be angry or to blow things off. We choose to judge people or to accept them. We choose to go forward or to live in the past. We choose to move forward and upward, or to stay stuck and stagnate.

The most critical choice we make, I believe, is how we choose to think. I read in Louise Hay's book that *"The only thing we are ever dealing with is a thought, and a thought can be changed."*

We *choose* to think negatively or to think positively.

If a negative thought pops into your mind, stop it right there and change it. If you are constantly thinking negative thoughts, change them. If something negative in your life is happening, change that. Don't give your power over to other people. That's giving them control over your life.

This is *your* life. Live it the way *you* choose to. Other people have their lives to live, so let them. You are responsible for living *yours*. It is up to you how it all turns out. Yes, there are some things you cannot control, but you can control how you *respond* to them. The way you respond can make all the difference in how your life plays out.

The key is to be aware. Be aware of what you are thinking and what you are doing. When you are aware, it gives you a moment to make a choice. Instead of just reacting to people and situations, stop your thought and watch yourself and what you are doing. Observe yourself as if you are starring in a movie.

When you step away and observe yourself you become aware of so much. It opens up your life and your options. If you are not aware and you react to something, you only get one option: your knee-jerk reaction. When you are aware, you can choose from a long list of options.

Be aware; be conscious. It'll change your life.

FORGIVENESS

Forgiveness is for *you*. Many people believe that it is something we are "supposed to do" for others. It is for others, too, but really, it sets *you* free. If you are harboring some anger, pain, or resentment toward another, it does much healing for your mind, heart, and soul to let it go. You can forgive someone without getting their acknowledgement or apology. It will still set you free.

One way to forgive someone is in person. Another way is to write a letter. You don't have to send it; in some situations, you may not even be able to. Journaling or expressing your feelings about the situation you perceive as wronging you is very therapeutic. You can write whatever you feel...the good, bad, and ugly. Write as much as you want and release it all. If you don't release it all in the first letter, write another later, and another if needed. The key is to release the anger, resentment, and pain so you can heal your own emotional wounds.

Once a letter has been written, you can mail it, rip it up, or burn it. It is important to take action to release your feelings and to let it go. Ripping or burning the letter is a way of taking physical action to release the pain from your mind, heart, and soul. Once the feelings have been released and physically let go, you may experience an inner peace. Letting go is the path to peace.

Three years ago, I forgave my father for perceived wrongs that happened throughout my childhood, teenage years, and adulthood. I had been holding on to that pain, anger, and resentment for forty-four years and it did nothing but cause me emotional stress. I forgave my father in person and received no apology. Once I realized that I may never receive an apology, I decided to really let it go.

I wrote him a letter. I did not send it. I read it out loud to myself to release any residual emotion and then burned it. I felt better, but it wasn't until I emailed him on Father's Day that I really let it go. I thanked him for all the positive things he had done for me in my life.

Once I forgave him, thanked him, and let it go, I was free...free to live my life without all that heavy baggage. I started to see the positive things he had done for me while I grew up. I began to understand him and where he was coming from. To this day, I see him with different eyes and appreciate what he went through while raising me. I now see that he did the best he could with the tools and knowledge he had at the time. Things look so different when you truly put yourself in someone else's shoes. Nothing can make that more real than actually being in a similar situation.

If you are harboring pain, anger or resentment toward another, do *yourself* some healing and forgive.

SELF-FORGIVENESS

Forgiving oneself is something that a lot of people don't think about. We tend to forgive others, but forget about ourselves and what we need. We need and deserve forgiveness just as much as anyone else does. You will feel worthy of your own forgiveness once you can do it. Forgiving yourself can help you to love yourself.

Maybe you've been in a toxic relationship and your partner was hurtful to you. Whether you stay in the relationship or not, it is healing to forgive the other person. It is even more healing to forgive yourself. If you do not forgive yourself, you are not loving yourself. Not forgiving yourself sends *you* the message that you are not worthy of forgiveness. You are telling yourself you are not lovable. You *are* worthy. You *are* lovable. You *do* deserve forgiveness. Forgiving yourself will help heal your emotional wounds. Forgiving yourself will help heal your life.

Forgiving yourself for allowing others to hurt you can be *very* therapeutic. Forgiving yourself for anything can be very healing.

APOLOGIES

Apologies are healing...when they are *authentic.* Authenticity is when someone is *truly* sincere. Both the giver and receiver then feel that there is true remorse for what was done. An authentic apology is believable and said with meaning. You know you've heard an authentic apology when someone apologizes for something and does not repeat the hurtful behavior.

If apologies are not authentic, we tend to continue to punish the person who did us wrong. Continual punishment does not heal the situation or the person; nor does an insincere apology.

Authentic apologies can heal broken hearts and emotional scars. I know; I experienced an extremely hurtful, degrading, and toxic relationship back in college. For years I harbored the emotional scars that it left.

Twenty years later, I received a letter from this man. All of the emotional pain came flooding back as if it had happened yesterday. I realized then that I had still been harboring anger, pain, and resentment.

Twenty years later, it was still there. Time had not erased the pain. We think we forget over time, because we are busy with life, but it can stay buried somewhere.

I realized I had not forgiven this man or released my pain. Not only that, but I realized he had not been aware of the damage he had done twenty years ago.

I wrote him a letter forgiving him for all of the verbal and emotional abuse I had experienced in our past relationship. I mentioned a few of the phrases he had said to me over and over and then forgave him for it. My forgiveness was authentic. I knew that in order for me to be free of the painful memory, I would need to be authentic in my forgiveness. I sent the letter and I was at peace. It didn't matter to me whether he received it or not. The important thing was that I wrote the letter to set myself free: free from anger, resentment, and painful memories. I thought that was it. Done. Free. Peace.

Three months later, I received a letter in reply. The letter was a page and a half long, but all I cared about was the one sentence that said, "I am *truly* sorry." In the letter he explained what type of person he had been back then and how he had taken steps to heal himself since.

I cried for twenty or thirty minutes after reading that letter. I realized how deep the pain had gone. I had believed that I had "let it go" after mailing him my letter of forgiveness. Little did I know how extremely healing it would feel to read his authentic apology. An authentic apology, in writing, had helped heal a pain inside that I had unknowingly been carrying around for twenty years. This was the most authentic and healing apology I had ever experienced. The last letter I sent was a letter of thanks. The man that I used to resent so much is now a man I respect.

If you've hurt someone and feel remorse, heal them. Apologize authentically.

LOSS OF A LOVED ONE

Loving others is a beautiful thing. Losing them is not. We become so attached to the ones we love that when it is time for them to go, it is a painful experience. We can cry, become angry, get depressed, eat comfort foods, drink, smoke, do drugs, fall into denial, or shut down emotionally. Coping with the experience can be a challenge.

If we are aware of the five stages of grief (denial, depression, anger, bargaining, and acceptance), we can hope to come through the situation with a little better understanding. At least it helps somewhat to know that others also go through these stages.

I know; I experienced loss at the death of my mother. She was the closest person I have ever known that has left my life. She was not only a beautiful woman, but also a beautiful soul. She was a great listener, a very perceptive and spiritual woman.

How do you let go of your mother…the person who brought you into the world? The one who taught you so many things as you were growing up; the person who listened to your problems and helped you to solve them, and also shared in your joys?

My mother left this world on January 29, 2009. She had so many health issues that I was happy to see her be rid of the pain. At the same time, I missed her so. Dealing with such conflicting emotions can be confusing and downright painful.

I knew the day was soon coming; yet when it happened, all I could say was, "No…No…No." It's as if my intellectual mind knew she was gone, yet my heart denied it. My mind told me that she was better off being out of pain, yet my heart was saying, "What about how I feel about losing my mother?" As I said: conflicting emotions.

The week of her death was a blur. The emotion, the family members, the funeral arrangements all blended together. Accepting reality was the toughest part. How was I supposed to deal with this? I had no manual to follow. The shock sets in and then, there you are…you and your emotions. Even if we think of healthy ways to cope, all of that seems to go out the window once the actual event happens.

I remember waking up the morning after she died and feeling like it had been a bad dream. My intellectual mind told me that it had happened, but my heart had not yet caught up to reality.

COPING MECHANISMS

To deal with the pain, I initially turned to unhealthy coping strategies. I drank, smoked, and consumed comfort foods, trying to numb the searing pain. I felt that if I numbed myself, somehow it wouldn't be true.

Using another coping technique, I found myself pushing away family members, friends and loved ones. Outside of work, I was alone, a lot. I did this to heal myself and also protect others from my pain, negativity, and depression. We all handle pain in our own way.

The coping mechanisms I tried were not all unhealthy. One healthy thing I did was to buy a house in the country. It was on five acres and surrounded by trees and nature. This became my healing place. I found myself driving an hour to work each way, five days a week, but I didn't care. Once I got home, it was worth it. It was always worth it to come home to a cozy five acres filled with healing trees and beautiful nature. Nature is always a great healer. It gives off healing energy and helps you to restore, recuperate, and recover.

Another healthy coping mechanism was talking. I did talk to people. It was helpful to express myself verbally. I found myself drawn to people who had lost someone dear to them. Expressing my feelings to them felt more comforting. It was as if they understood. Discussing loss actually brought us closer in the relationship. It's as if it created a new bond that was not there before. Expressing how you feel to other people can be very therapeutic, whether it be friends, family or a counselor.

I cried, and still cry today, about my mother being gone. Sometimes I feel the pain will never go away. There just seem to be longer gaps between crying sessions. Crying can be a very therapeutic way of releasing a wide range of emotions including anger, grief, depression or pain. Releasing this emotion is beneficial to anyone who may be holding in unexpressed feelings. If you are uncomfortable crying front of others, find a time and place to get away from people.

Another healthy thing I did was talk to God. When I did not feel like talking to people, I talked to God...many, many, times. He became my best friend. There were times when I yelled, screamed and cried out of anger and emotional pain. Sometimes I yelled and screamed at God. No matter how angry or upset I became, He was there for me, listening, accepting me as I was, loving me. Although it was the most painful time, the experience brought me closer to God than ever before.

A friend's mother once told me that crying is "cleansing to the soul." In my self-growth trainings someone mentioned that the act of crying was the ice melting off your heart. Another person said that when you release negative or painful emotions, you make more space in your heart for love and joy to enter. Do your body, mind and spirit some good. Have a good cry, you'll feel much better.

Journaling is also a great way to release and heal. It was for me. The thing about journaling is you get the thoughts and feelings out. When they are in your head, they keep bouncing around inside with nowhere to go. You keep feeling and experiencing them over and over again, until they are released outside your heart and mind. With journaling, you really do release the feelings, thoughts, and pain. You can write whatever you want, whenever you want, however you want. You can scream, shout, cry, and get angry on paper and it's okay.

In fact, journaling can pull out some of the emotion that you may have been holding on to. One technique that I have found helpful is to write it all out and then read it out loud to yourself. That's when I feel more emotion come out. And that's what we need to do: get it out. Holding on to unresolved or unexpressed emotion can only grow like a cancer within you that you end up processing over and over again. Getting it out is the path to peace.

I know, because my mother was very good at holding in her emotions. She did not like confrontation. She was so sweet, kind, and sensitive that she never wanted to hurt anyone or make them feel uncomfortable. So she held in her emotions to protect *their* feelings. That sounds great—like a thoughtful, considerate thing to do—but really, she ended up hurting herself, day after day, year after year. It got to the point where her unreleased feelings built up and started to come out through physical ailments. If she was going to hold on to those emotions year after year, then her body was going to speak for her.

I believe her body was trying to tell her to release her feelings. If she didn't, her body would get sicker and sicker. I have learned a great deal from my mother. This was one of the big lessons: to express myself. Just like Madonna says: *"Express yourself."* If you don't, you will pay a price.

I was not a fan of confrontation either. So I held in my feelings for years. The day came when I could no longer do that. I also came to realize that I had been making everyone else's feelings more important than mine. It was a self-worth issue I had. Once I got into therapy, I realized I had learned this behavior (a coping mechanism) from my mother. I also learned that my feelings were just as important as anyone else's. I deserved to be able to express myself just as other people did. When I learned that it was healthy to express myself, I decided to continue.

Now, you can express your feelings in a healthy responsible way, or in an irresponsible way. We all need to be responsible about the way we express our feelings. If we are not, we must be prepared for the consequences.

As a personal trainer and fitness instructor, over the years I have learned to tell people to listen to their bodies. I would say to my clients and class participants, "If you don't listen to your body, it will whisper to you. If you don't listen, it will talk to you. If you don't listen, it will yell at you. If you don't listen, it will scream at you. If you don't listen, it will cry."

My mother's body got to the point where it cried. And then she died. She listened to her body, but what she was not listening to were her feelings. She was not listening to the message that her feelings needed to be expressed.

Listening to your feelings is also important. Expressing them is a healthy way of expressing who you are and how you feel. Listen to your body, but also listen to your feelings. When something is coming up within you, let it out. It comes up for a reason: to get out.

When I went to various intense group therapy trainings in Dallas, a lot of emotion would come up. After forty years of holding in my emotions, a lot came up. So much came up and out, it was as if I were vomiting. I coined a phrase while going through these trainings—I call it "emotional puking." It doesn't sound pretty, but it sure feels great after it's out. As I've said, getting it out is the path to peace.

REAL THERAPY

There are many different approaches to taking a look at yourself. These can range from hard-core therapy and workshops to exercises like mirror work or journaling. Everyone has a different preference and comfort level for what they are able to do. Some people may wish to take it slow and easy, experiencing steady progress; others may be on a mission and go for it hard and fast. The bigger steps you take, the greater and quicker the rewards. Not everyone is cut out for the hard-core, determined path. Some people are very sensitive and feel more comfortable learning in small increments.

Eight years ago, I received my "therapy wake-up call," from an ex-boyfriend. He was extremely critical and wore me down time and time again. I felt drained and exhausted after talking to him on the phone for only a few minutes. There would be times when I was happy and energetic, only to feel like a deflated balloon after talking to him. I grew tired of the arguing, insecurity, and constant criticism.

Stress had been eating away at me for months. I was working full time, which included *extreme* amounts of intense physical exercise, being a single parent to my seven-year-old daughter, and tolerating my controlling and critical boyfriend. My fitness job was draining me physically. My daughter, who needed me, was draining me emotionally, and my boyfriend drained me with constant criticism.

To escape or numb the stress, I turned to wine. Before I knew it, I was drinking four or five nights a week. Some nights it was just one glass of wine, other times it was a bottle. I reached a point where something had to give.

My daughter was staying and I was not going to quit my job. The boyfriend had to go. Breaking up with him was a challenge. It was my first experience with a roller-coaster relationship. Every time I broke it off with him, somehow I allowed him to talk me back in. It was dysfunctional. After hearing the constant criticism, I started to believe it. And I must admit, there was some truth to it. He told me some things about myself that I did not want to see or hear.

I chose to go to therapy for the first time, not because I was "crazy," but because I was tired of experiencing disappointing and unfulfilling relationships. I made a decision to take a good look at myself. Making that decision did not happen overnight. I struggled with the thought of going to a counselor, because I have a degree in Psychology. Getting past my ego and the thought that I should know how to do this, took a bit of time. I came to realize, that maybe I was too close to the situation in my relationships and an outsider might be able to see what I was not seeing.

Some people feel uncomfortable talking about their personal life with a total stranger, but I saw it as a relief. I could talk to this person about what I thought were "failures."

The "failures" were actually learning experiences.

There was comfort in the fact that I would feel less embarrassed telling someone that I did not know, rather than someone I did know.

ONE-ON-ONE THERAPY: EMDR

I tried one therapist for two sessions and did not feel I was getting much out of it, but shortly after that, someone recommended a different therapist and a type of therapy called EMDR. I was intrigued. EMDR is designed to be fast and effective. I did not want to end up on a "couch" talking for years and paying thousands of dollars, like people do in some forms of therapy. EMDR worked well for me.

My EMDR therapy used handheld vibrating items that helped me to relax during meditation and affirmations that were guided by a qualified therapist. The vibrating item was supposed to relax me as I expressed my feelings. I did feel relaxed, even when speaking about past experiences that were upsetting; it made them easier to talk about. There were times when I was angry and used profanity, and there were times when I simply cried. After releasing my feelings, I felt an inner peace and calmness. At that point, I repeated affirmations that my therapist said out loud. I continued to do this until the anger, crying, or emotion passed.

Feeling the effectiveness of EMDR, I continued the therapy twice a week for five months. It was effective because of the mission I was on: to heal myself. I was determined to see what it was about myself that kept leading me down the same path in relationships. The therapy helped me release some of my childhood experiences. Little did I know that working toward emotional health is like peeling the layers of an onion, and that I had so far only peeled the first layer.

I was happy to purge the negative feelings of the past. The boyfriend that had "criticized me" into therapy—who was unwilling to go himself—was actually "therapied" right out of my life. So, he may have been "right" about some things, but he was also purged along with my negative childhood experiences. In this case, "being right" for him meant losing me and the relationship.

To this day, I thank him. I have thanked him in person. My eyes have been opened and it's interesting to see that maybe he could have benefited from some therapy. Like I said, none of us are perfect.

We all have our issues to deal with, in our own time. The longer we go without facing them, the longer we stay in pain.

GROUP THERAPY TRAINING

Group therapy training is a useful tool to help people see themselves through the eyes of others. This form of therapy is straightforward and is about being honest with yourself and others. One–on-one therapy in a private office is useful in its own way, but group therapy helps us to hear what others see in us and in our behavior. It is sometimes harder to face a group of people and their opinions than it is to face one person. It can be intense, yet very effective.

Although my life was going well for a while, I reached a point where I wanted something more. The first section of the group training I did was five ten- to twelve-hour days long. I had no idea what I was getting myself into. It was intense, yet I was intrigued. I feel that the intensity of the training helped me to purge more emotion at a quicker rate. It was very successful. One reason it was successful was my open-mindedness and determination to "see" myself.

The first training led to more trainings over the next three or four years. I did a training session when I felt I needed one. There were times when I was not interested, but other times when I felt an urge to move forward with my emotional health.

In group trainings, I got to see how others saw me. It was eye-opening. The trainings helped me to see myself and others in a way I had never seen before. To this day, I am much more honest with myself. When I am being dishonest, I tend to catch myself in the process and "wake myself up" to the truth.

PET THERAPY

Whether it is a cat, dog, horse, or hamster, animals heal us. They help lower our blood pressure, decrease stress, and bring joy to our hearts. They don't give us unwanted advice, criticism, or judgmental comments. Pets don't care if we are tall, short, fat, beautiful, ugly, or something in between. They don't care what job we have or what car we drive. Pets make us feel safe—safe to say whatever is on our minds, safe to cry, and safe to love. And they love us back.

EQUINE THERAPY

Equine therapy involves horses and people working together to create a variety of things. It could be self-growth, self-discovery, team-building, or psychotherapy. Horses cannot be fooled. As humans, we can go around trying to be something we are not, acting different from the way we really feel, or just plain lie to ourselves and everyone around us...everyone except horses. As the famous horse trainer Chris Irwin would say, "Horses don't lie."

Because horses can't be fooled, they are so valuable in self-growth, self-discovery, team-building, and therapy. They not only see past our false fronts, they also mirror our behavior. They let us know when we are being real and when we are not. Many therapists and horse trainers are working together to help make people aware of their own behavior, giving insight and healing to many people across the world.

Horses...in my life? They've been a love of my life since I was a child. I used to watch cowboy and Indian movies with my father, always feeling sorry for the poor horses in battle that were injured or went down. In grade school I went through horse book after horse book, reading, studying, and drawing the various kinds of horses. My toys were realistic, plastic horses. In art class I drew horse picture after horse picture. My first major purchase with my own money was a pair of Frye cowboy boots...and I have been wearing cowboy hats since I was seventeen years old.

When people would ask me what I wanted to be when I grew up, I would say, "I would like to live on a ranch and raise horses." I begged and pleaded with my parents to buy me a horse, but it never happened. Years later, when I was in my thirties, my father told me that the reason they didn't get me a horse was because I was approaching the age of being interested in boys and they thought I would not take care of a horse. Looking back, I think they had it backwards. Getting me a horse probably would have kept me busy and delayed my interest in boys… but who's really to know? I was always drawn to Palominos back then and dreamed of owning one.

At age forty-six, I decided to spend a week at a friend's guest ranch in Bandera, Texas. It was the week of Christmas; my daughter was spending it with her father and I was doing what I could to cope with my first Christmas without my mother. I decided to give myself a gift of time on a ranch: a place to relax, to be around horses, and hoped that being in that environment would be healing to my heart. Not only was it healing to my heart, but it was also healing to my soul…something I was not expecting.

Although I paid full price for that week as a guest, I chose to work the ranch with the wranglers—to live life on a ranch, to experience it for *real*. I woke up at 6:00 a.m. and headed for the stables. I fed the horses, turned them out, brushed them, and helped take guests out on trail rides for a week.

One day, while feeding one of the Palominos an apple, I started talking to him. His name was Ike. Out of all the horses on the ranch, including three Palominos, I was drawn to Ike. I'd pet him and talk to him and at one point, I started to cry right there in the stall with him. I hugged him, loved on him, and cried my eyes out…not sure where it was coming from. Was I missing my mother? Or was I healing an old childhood wound…a long, lost dream that had not yet materialized?

As I cried alongside Ike, one of the tough and abrasive wranglers walked up and saw me. We had joked around with one another that week and he couldn't figure out why I was being emotional. He, who had been around horses all his life, thought it was silly for me to cry with a horse. I wiped my eyes and told him that it would be difficult for him to understand, considering that he had been around horses all his life while I had not. I told him about my childhood dream that had never been realized. He looked at me with a neutral face and said, "Come here." I followed him to the tack room and he handed me some apple horse treats and a brush and said in an ice-melting-off-his-heart kind of way, "Go ahead...brush him."

After I was done brushing and bonding with Ike, I told the wrangler that I was going to my cabin to shower. He looked at me with this not-sure-what-to-do look and said, "All right, but no more bawling!" He was a tough and abrasive cowboy...with a heart. That day, we became friends.

My point is, horses are very healing animals. They are nonjudgmental, unconditionally loving, and spiritual. That horse helped me to release pent-up emotion that needed to be let go...to be healed.

So, I didn't get a horse when I was a child, but I got to live on a ranch, experience working it, and to bond with a Palomino named Ike. That was the best Christmas gift I could have given myself. At an emotionally difficult time in my life and experiencing my first Christmas without my mother, I chose to put myself in an environment that not only helped heal the loss I felt, but also helped to heal my inner child.

This was not the "traditional" Christmas that I was used to. It was a unique Christmas that I spent with a new "family"...a ranch family and a horse named Ike. It was an extremely healing Christmas. Thanks, Ike. (See Resource section in back of book for equine therapy and workshop sources).

JOURNALING

Some people feel more comfortable talking to someone. Others feel more comfortable writing. The act of writing can be very therapeutic.

Journaling can express our reactions to experiences. It can counteract the negative effects of stress and decrease the symptoms of many health conditions, improve our cognitive functioning, and strengthen our immune system.

Journaling is a very valuable tool to help us express feelings that we may otherwise not express. It is a safe place to put our feelings and to "get them out." Journaling helps us realize what we feel, how we feel, and why we feel it. Writing it out helps us to see things in the third person and to recognize things we may not normally notice. When thoughts are floating around in our head, we are too close to them and there may be a pattern that is difficult to interrupt. Once the thoughts are written down, we can see them for what they *are*—not what they *seem* to be.

Journaling can be whatever you want it to be. You can write anything you want, how you want, whenever you want. You can yell, scream or cry on paper: it's safe. Some people journal to express their feelings whenever they feel them, while others write down what they did just to keep a record of what happened. Journaling can help you release anything that you may feel a need to get out.

Other benefits to journaling are that it's private, and that the pen and paper do not judge you. Many people put things on paper they would never tell anyone else. There is a sense of freedom when you release something you've been holding in. Getting it out is the path to peace. Journaling can heal us.

GRATITUDE JOURNALING

Gratitude journaling is exactly what it sounds like: writing about whatever you are grateful for. Being grateful is one thing, but *writing* about your gratitude is quite powerful. Gratitude journaling is uplifting, encouraging, and makes you feel wonderful.

You could make a list of things you are grateful for, or you could write the way you feel about your blessings in sentence form. Gratitude journaling takes you to a place of appreciation. No matter how bad things may appear, they could always be worse. There is always someone out there who has it worse than you.

Have you ever been upset about having a bad day and then later talk to someone who is in a much worse situation than you are? It definitely makes you feel lucky, blessed, and grateful for what you *do* have. All of a sudden, your "bad" day gets put into perspective and you realize your "bad" day isn't so bad. It may even appear good next to someone else's situation.

Getting into the habit of writing about gratitude daily will make all the difference in the world. It not only changes how you see things, but it can change your life. Gratitude journaling for a day can help you improve how you see things that day. Doing it on a *daily basis* can improve how you see everything *on a regular basis*. As I said before, *"The only thing we are ever dealing with is a thought, and a thought can be changed.* Change your thoughts, change your life." (Louise Hay.)

Next time you are feeling down, angry, or upset, try gratitude journaling. I guarantee that it will make you feel better and your life better.

SOUL JOURNALING

Soul journaling is writing from your soul. It starts with listening to your soul and then putting what you hear on paper.

Sometimes just writing about anything can be a beginning. Usually when we start out writing, it is about things that are bothering us. It is usually the *ego mind* that is complaining or being negative. Once the writing continues and the emotions start flowing, you notice a turn in the direction of your writing. That's the *soul* stepping in: when you get deep and you come to "aha!" moments. You come to realizations that you were not aware of before. You see that the original paragraph of writing was about some surface, mundane thing, but by the end of your writing you find that your ego is gone and your soul has appeared.

When you get to the *soul* journaling part, keep it going. Don't stop, let it flow. Don't worry about messiness, spelling, or punctuation. That's not what's important. The thoughts, feeling, and realizations, are what are important.

Soothe your soul. Do some soul journaling.

REAL POSITIVE ATTITUDE & EMOTIONAL HEALING

Keeping a positive attitude makes all the difference when combining other healthy habits. Studies have been done about attitude with proper nutrition and exercise. Neither one tends to keep a person *real healthy* without positivity.

MIRROR WORK

The mirror reflects much about the way we look. It helps us apply makeup, remove something from an eye, and see cars to the rear and side of us while driving. It also helps us to view, up close, any and all physical flaws.

The mirror can be an enemy, or it can be a friend. Looking at yourself in the mirror does not only reveal physical aspects, assets, and imperfections, it can also reveal your emotional soul. Have you ever looked into the mirror to see your *emotional self?*

It's a whole other world.

Mirror work is something I learned from Louise Hay. Ms. Hay experienced a very traumatic life growing up. She was abused physically, verbally, emotionally, and sexually. Over the years, she found a way to heal her emotional wounds. Not only did she heal her emotions, she healed her life and helped many others heal theirs. She has written many books which range from healing yourself and your life to healing your body. One book in particular that I found helpful was *I Can Do It*. It is a small book filled with affirmations.

Louise recommends using affirmations to change our thoughts. When we change our thoughts, we change our lives. Ridding our minds of negative thoughts can only do us good. When we think negatively, we get negativity. When we think positively, we get positivity. Louise found that if you say affirmations with emotion, they work. If you say them with *a lot* of emotion, they work even better.

We've all heard of affirmations. You know: they are statements you say out loud to help you think positively. Affirmations are a great way to train your brain to think differently. Some say that positive affirmations work and some say they don't. Why the discrepancy? Why would affirmations work for some and not for others? The first time I tried saying affirmations, I had a difficult time believing them as I said them. I wanted to believe, but I felt I was lying to myself. How was I supposed to change my life with affirmations when I didn't believe they were true? Well, for starters, affirmations tend to work much better if you believe them. Repeating an affirmation with *feeling* gives it more power, which makes it more effective.

If you don't believe the affirmation, try thinking of it in a different way. Find a way to believe it. For example, the affirmation "I am money" may not be believable due to the small amount of money you have in the bank. Think of the affirmation in a *different* way, such as "I am money" (because of my gifts and talents). If you think about it, you are paid money at your job because of the gifts, talents and skills that you bring to the job. If you *leave* the job, you take your gifts, talents and skills *with you*, therefore you take the *money* (your gifts and talents) with you, to the next job. You will "be money" at the next job because you bring *your* gifts, talent and skills to the new job. Therefore, *you are money*.

In her book, Louise takes affirmations a step further. Instead of just saying them out loud or writing them, like most people do, Louise recommends that you say them in the mirror while looking yourself in the eye (hence the term "mirror work"). Saying an affirmation ten times is great, but saying it while looking yourself in the eye creates a whole new magic. It reaches down into your soul.

After repeating the affirmation several times, you may notice some emotion coming up that may otherwise not surface. Getting the emotion to come up is good. As I say, it's about getting it out. Once it's out, you have room in your heart for love, joy, and peace. Keep looking yourself in the eye as you say the affirmation and let the emotion come, then let it go. If tears come, keep repeating the affirmation and keep looking yourself in the eye until the tears stop.

Once the tears stop, you will feel an inner peace. This is a form of self-therapy. It helps you reach down into your soul and release any and all emotional wounds that may have been covered up for years. These can be anything from feelings of being unloved since childhood to emotional issues you have with money.

Not all affirmations will bring up emotion. It all depends on how consistent you are in using affirmations and where your soul is in the healing process. I have found that one affirmation will bring up no emotion one day and then bring a flood of tears the next time. There have been times when I said a certain affirmation ten times on a Sunday and nothing came up, yet saying it on Tuesday brought up a load of emotion. It is an amazing process. One day an affirmation is said with total confidence, and the next day it is said with sadness, tears, and pain. If you don't feel any emotion after repeating the affirmation ten times, don't worry. Just say it like you mean it. Maybe there isn't a wound there to heal...or maybe it's just not ready to be healed today.

What I have done in the past is to repeat the affirmation as the emotion comes up. I may say it ten times or I may say it twenty—it all depends on when the emotion subsides. My goal has always been to say it over and over until there are no more tears left to cry about that particular affirmation or thought. I have found that saying it over and over until I stop crying actually helps release residual emotion that might be left inside. (I have done the same thing with music. I have listened to a song that brings up emotion and played it over and over until there are no more tears to cry. This is with *healing* music, not negative, depressing music that tortures you emotionally.)

One of the affirmations I've found to be very effective is "I am love." This affirmation sticks in my memory due to the amount of feeling and emotion I felt while saying it to myself in the mirror. Saying these affirmations while looking yourself in the eye is about being truly honest with yourself. You'll know whether you believe it or not as you say it. Say it at least ten times, and really look yourself in the eye. Don't make it a robotic experience. Say it like you mean it. Saying affirmations with meaning triggers something deep inside of you. If nothing comes up, move on to the next affirmation. Don't give up on that particular affirmation, though; it may trigger some emotion another day. Just make sure you choose affirmations that you are *drawn to.* If the affirmation subject feels right, but the wording doesn't, then change the wording until it feels right for you.

The mirror work technique is not only therapeutic and effective, it's also very easy, very healing, and inexpensive. I think of it as "free therapy." It can help heal emotional wounds and set you free. All you need is a mirror, some affirmations, and your eyes...the window to your soul.

Try it. Pick a mirror, look yourself in the eye, and say, "I love you." You may feel silly at first, but if you're alone, who cares? It's about the healing and the peace you receive afterwards.

*Note: *Doing mirror work in a private, safe space is recommended.*

REAL ENERGY HEALING

CHAKRA HEALING

Chakras are areas of energy in the body. There are seven main chakras and many other small ones. The seven main chakras are in development from birth until we are thirty years old. Each represents a different category of development: the base chakra, sacral chakra, solar plexus chakra, heart chakra, throat chakra, brow chakra, and the crown chakra.

THE SEVEN MAIN CHAKRAS AND DEVELOPMENTAL STAGES ARE:

Base: 0–4 years of age
Sacral: 4–8 years
Solar Plexus: 8–12 years
Heart: 12–16 years
Throat: 16–21 years
Brow: 21–26 years
Crown: 26–30 years

When a person experiences any type of trauma (physical or emotional) during these seven stages between birth and age thirty, certain areas of a person's being may be lacking. A person's chakra centers repeat every thirty years, giving opportunity to heal and center on what may be in need of healing. Chakras can be healed or balanced by doing various healing exercises and meditations or by receiving help from a chakra therapist. (See Chakra Energy Vortex Chart in Appendix).

MOTIVATION

Motivation is about doing. Being sedentary or lethargic only keeps us stuck. If you're happy where you are in life, then stay there. If not, get up. Do something. If you want a change in your life, do something different.

If you want to have a healthy body, eat healthy foods. If you don't feel like it, focus on the thought of how you will feel *after* you eat something healthy. Really absorb the feeling of how good your body will feel and how proud you'll feel about yourself.

If you want to lose weight, get up and exercise. Even just walking is exercise. If you don't feel like it, focus on the thought of how good you will feel *after* you are done exercising. Really think about how energized you'll be and how proud you'll feel about yourself.

Procrastination can be a challenge to overcome. Once again, it comes back to your thoughts. *The only thing you are ever dealing with is a thought, and a thought can be changed.* Think about how good you will feel *after* getting the task done. Besides, once you get started on the project, it's usually not nearly as bad as we originally thought it would be. The thought was worse than the reality…and, once again, a thought can be changed.

VISUALIZATION

Visualization can change your life. I have used this technique many times. It's amazing how powerful our minds are if we use them in a positive way.

Visualization can bring us what we'd like to have in our lives. Visualization is about focusing on what we *do* want in life, not what we don't want. When we visualize what we'd like to have, over and over again, it begins to come about. We can manifest anything we'd like. The challenge is to keep that in mind continuously.

I have visualized anything from being lean and healthy to getting a new job that I wanted. All I did was visualize myself getting the phone call about the new job, going to the new office in my new job clothes, interacting with the new people and seeing myself enjoying the job immensely. It's amazing how many times it has come to be for me.

The key, once again, is your thoughts. Keeping your thoughts positive can change your life. If you start to think negatively, that's ok, change it! Replace it with a positive thought. Remember, *the only thing we are ever dealing with is a thought, and a thought can be changed.* Visualization is a thought on top of a thought on top of a thought.

Just make the thoughts positive!

Note: *The more detail you put into your visualization, the more effective it will be.*

REAL POSITIVE ENVIRONMENT

Surrounding ourselves with a positive environment can make all the difference in the world. When our environment is positive, it helps support a positive attitude. Our environment includes the earth we live on and the home we live in.

FENG SHUI

Feng shui came from China thousands of years ago. It was originally designed to help grow better crops, which were set up in a certain direction for best results. After succeeding with crop placement, the Chinese applied placement design to the home.

The two schools of feng shui are Compass School and Form School. The Compass school uses direction (north, south, east, and west) and the homeowner's birth information, while the Form school uses a grid that is laid over the floor plan of a home or office. You can also apply feng shui to your yard, desk, and many other places.

Feng shui has an intriguing way of helping you manifest positive things in your life by creating positive chi (energy) within your home. After making various changes to create positive chi (energy), it's only a matter of days, weeks, (sometimes a few months) before other positive changes start taking place. It's not just about rearranging furniture. It enhances various areas of your life by helping you focus on what you *do* want, not what you don't want. Feng shui can help you improve your health, wealth, career, relationships, and more. All of these improvements can be done by changing a few things in your home. It is fun, simple and easy to apply.

THINGS TO KEEP IN MIND WHEN APPLYING FENG SHUI IN YOUR HOME:

*Live with what you love
*Aim for safety and comfort
*Simplify and organize

Feng shui can also help you to detox your environment, which starts with decluttering your home. Some people have a difficult time getting rid of things they don't really need. Before getting rid of an item, ask yourself these questions:

Do I love it?

Do I use it?

Does it give me a good feeling when I look at it?

If you love it, keep it. If you use it, keep it. If it gives you a good feeling, keep it.

If anything is broken, fix it or get rid of it. If you don't love it or use it, get rid of it.

As a feng shui consultant, I have experienced many positive changes in my life, from getting a job I wanted to creating a love relationship. I have even feng shui-ed someone *out* of my life! Sounds crazy, but it's true. I have also seen what feng shui can do for others when they are open to it. I have helped people increase income, be rid of a lawsuit, and bring love into their lives.

REAL SOUL ACTIVITIES

MEDITATION

Meditation is a great way to reduce stress, lower blood pressure, and center yourself. Moving or sitting meditation can both be effective, depending on your personality, your goals, and what works for you. I, personally, am not very good at sitting meditation…yet. I admire those who can sit and meditate every morning and every evening for thirty minutes or more. I hadn't had much luck until I tried various moving meditations. Not all meditations have to be sitting still or lying down. You can relax, think, resolve issues, sort out feelings and situations while doing a moving meditation.

Some of these are hiking, running, painting, yard work, yoga, meditation walks in a labyrinth, being out in nature and meditation stretch class. My meditation stretch class is a Serenity Stretch class where I do a short meditation at the end of class. The meditation only lasts about seven to ten minutes, but it is very effective in relaxing my body, mind, and spirit. Remember, it is *Real healthy* to slow down now and then, or even to stop for a few minutes.

LABYRINTH MEDITATION WALK

A labyrinth is an ancient symbol that relates to wholeness. It is a type of walkway or path that looks like a maze. It is different from a maze, however, since it leads you to the center with only one way in and one way out. The walk into the labyrinth represents a path to our own center: to go within. The walk out of it represents going back out into the world.

The two most common labyrinths are the Chartres and the Classic-7. The Chartres was built in Chartres Cathedral in France around 1201 AD. It has eleven circuits and four quadrants. The Classic-7 design is simpler and goes as far back as 1500 BC. The design is found on ancient coins from the island of Crete, so the labyrinth design is often called Cretan. The Cretan or Classic-7 design has seven circuits.

The labyrinth is a path of meditation, prayer, joy, or appreciation. It helps you unwind or release anything that may be on your mind. It is usually walked in silence, but it can also be a walk of joy accompanied with music, or done in other ways. Most people find the labyrinth very calming.

One way to walk the labyrinth is to choose what you want to focus on prior to the walk. After choosing your subject of focus, you may choose an item to represent the subject of focus. This item may be a rock, a stick, an acorn, a coin, or some other personal item that has significance to you or your meditation subject. Once you choose your item, you may walk the labyrinth as fast or as slow as you like. Take as much time as you need.

Once you arrive at the center of the labyrinth, you may say a prayer, meditate, or focus on whatever it is you'd like to get from the experience. After your prayer or meditation, feel free to leave your meditation item in the center. When you feel it is time, slowly turn from the center and reverse the path you came in on.

Many people walk to the center of the labyrinth with a concern on their mind and feel a release once meditating in the center. Some people feel a release after prayer and setting down the chosen item in the center. Others feel a release on the walk out of the labyrinth. It can be very therapeutic to "let go" while exiting the labyrinth. Most people find walking the labyrinth healing and relaxing. Whatever your intention, know that it is *your* experience while walking the labyrinth. Some people choose to walk the labyrinth alone; others choose to walk with a group. It's up to you to choose whatever experience you desire. The main thing is to focus on that experience.

There is no right or wrong way to walk a labyrinth. If you've never done it and would like some guidance, you may want to keep the following in mind:

Before the walk: Gather your intentions (mental, spiritual or emotional thoughts) or items to symbolize your focus, subject, or intent (rock, twig, acorn, coin or personal item).

During the walk to the center: Take time to focus on the meditation subject, intention, or prayer, or release all concerns of the mind.

At the center for meditation, prayer, or peace: Spend time in the center meditating, praying, or experiencing centering or inner peace.

Exiting the center: Reverse your path, using the time to reflect, relax, release, and think about how it will all unfold or be applied to your life.

Closing: Meditate, say a prayer of gratitude, or just reflect on the entire labyrinth experience once you are outside the labyrinth. This represents your outside life, the world of everyday experience.

My labyrinth experience has been with the Classic-7. I created my own Classic-7 labyrinth in a secluded, cozy, wooded area on my land. I enjoy it immensely. It is simple to use, relaxing to walk, and beneficial to my mind, body, and spirit.

SOUL PAINTING

Painting can be a very therapeutic type of moving meditation. It gives your mind a break from the world and life's "have-to's." To use this kind of moving meditation, you can create a masterpiece on canvas or just change the color of the walls in your bedroom.

VISION BOARDS

Vision boarding helps you put your visions, dreams, and goals on paper, in writing, and in picture form. You gather pictures and/or words from magazines and create a picture or collage of them. It's another way of writing down your goals but with a different approach. This is a way to be creative, put your goals in motion, or manifest what it is you'd like to see happen in your life. Vision boards help make a statement to the universe about what direction you'd like your life to go.

So, if you want to get your vision, dreams, and goals up and moving, move them with a vision board. Get your magazines, scissors, and glue. I like to put on some relaxing music on while doing my vision boards. It is a very peaceful way to put positive energy toward your dreams.

After you've completed your board, make sure you place it somewhere where you will see it often—for instance, on your bathroom by the mirror or by your front door. This way you see it often and think about it, putting positive thoughts and energy toward your dreams. Every time you brush your teeth, you see that vision board. Every time you walk out the door to go somewhere, you see that vision board and you are reminded of what you *do* want in your life. Every time you look or think about that vision board, you reinforce the positive energy that helps to create your vision.

It works. I have had several dreams fulfilled since doing boards. They may not manifest overnight or within a week, but be patient; it *does* work. Look at the board, think about your goals. After a month or two, move the vision board to a new location. This way, you start to see it all over again. We tend to stop seeing things in our environment when they are in the same spot day after day. Why do you think retail stores change their merchandise around so much? So that we will see it—or "re-see" it.

Think up a vision, create a dream, and make a goal. Visualize it. Dream it. Cut it out. Paste it. Create it. Post it. Look at it. Manifest it. Enjoy it.

Soul Boards

Soul boarding is the same thing as vision boarding, except the focus is on what you feel your soul desires. Create a collage about your soul's path: what you *feel* (not think) the path is.

Gratitude Boards

A Gratitude Board is...you guessed it, almost the same as vision boarding, but it focuses on what you are *grateful* for in your life.

PHOTO BOARDS

Photo boards are collages made with personal photos. Most people have at least one drawer or box of photos from the past that are just sitting there, doing nothing. The photos are in your possession, but not being used or displayed in any way.

When I lived in Atlanta years ago, I got out my big box of personal photographs that had been stored away. I didn't want to throw them out, but I didn't feel they were being of use. I decided to make some collages with them.

When Mother's Day came around, I made a collage for my mother. I selected all of my favorite photos of us together from childhood through adulthood. To see my mother's face when she opened the gift was priceless. I received the joy of making the collage, and she received a heartfelt gift of memories that she could display in her home.

For Christmas, I made several collages for family members. I did the same for Father's Day, my friends' birthdays, and more. Before I knew it, I had used many of the photos in sentimental pieces of artwork.

I displayed collages of my daughter from when she was a baby and also did a collage of my life. I selected photos of myself as a baby, toddler, teenager and up through adulthood. It sounds like just an art project, but I was surprised to experience therapeutic effects from just going through old photos and creating a timeline of my life. It helped me remember old memories, sort out various things about my life and all I had experienced. The project was relaxing, but also healing.

So, if you have a bunch of old photos just sitting around doing nothing, take some time for yourself and create a gift, a piece of art, or relive some memories. Giving the photo boards to friends and family is not only relaxing and therapeutic for you, but also brings a warm fuzzy feeling to those you love. They will cherish the thought, time, and energy you put into this sentimental gift.

JOURNALING

Whether you use *gratitude journaling*, *soul journaling* or simply keep a journal where you write your goals, dreams and affirmations, *journaling* is a great soul activity. (Please see previous sections on journaling under Therapy, and the journaling handouts in the Appendix.)

CREATING

Creating is a process that soothes the soul and makes you feel powerful. Taking nothing and making it into something brings a feeling that sticks with you. There is a feeling of productivity and a sense of pride when you have completed your creation. Creating can be painting your living room, cooking a beautiful meal, or starting a new business. It doesn't matter what you create, as long as it is something that you love to do.

I know I am at my happiest when I am creating something. I am in the moment and I lose track of time. When I lose track of time, I know I'm in my element. Creating, for me, can be writing a book, making a vision board, or feng shui-ing my home. When I am on a creative roll, I can go for hours not thinking about yesterday or tomorrow. What a relaxing place to be! Creating gives you a project that you are passionate about and helps you break free from worries and concerns over what happened yesterday or what you have to do tomorrow. The soul loves to create. We are all creators and we can create anything we like. Do something for your soul—create something.

MUSIC

Music...what would we do without music? Music is so powerful. It can lift us up, bring us down, help us to relive old memories, or heal our souls. Music can make us dance or help us relax.

I did a project for a music therapy class years ago and I was amazed at the effect it had on me and my emotions. I played all different types of music in a one- to two-hour period. I went from happy and dancing to slow and relaxed, remembering times in high school and reliving old relationships. My emotions were all over the place. The beautiful thing about music is the variety of it all. There are types of music that are great for relaxing, dancing, remembering, creating, and releasing emotion.

If you are in a bad mood, put on some happy, upbeat music. If you are wound up and want to relax, put on some soothing music. If you want to reminisce, put on some oldies. The list is endless. Just know that music can help shift your mood.

There was a time when I played a particular song every morning before I left for work. This song was so upbeat and lifted me up and into a great mood every day. I noticed that the days I played that song before leaving the house, I had a great day. The days I forgot, or skipped playing the song, were not as uplifting for me. Playing a song before you start your day can make all the difference in the world. A song only lasts for three or four minutes and you can find time for that as you get ready to leave the house.

Next time you want to experience a soul activity, put on some music that you love. Your heart will sing and your soul will dance!

SOUL DANCING

Soul dancing is about letting go—of your worries, concerns and stress. Dancing in a club, dance hall, or just in your own living room can take you to a different place.

When I go dancing, I dance my butt off. I dance off stress, frustration, or negativity. Dancing is not only fun, but also a great release. It takes you to a place where no one knows. You can lose yourself and be in the moment. When you are in the moment, the rest of the world goes away. Let's be real; sometimes that is a beautiful thing.

If you are embarrassed to "let go" in public while on the dance floor, then use your living room. The living room is just as fun and much more private. Dancing in private allows you to lose all inhibitions and move however you like. I love the phrase, "Dance like no one is watching." My mother gave me a plaque with that saying on it for

Christmas many years ago. I love it, display in my home, and always try to remember to "let go" and dance like no one is watching.

Do some soul dancing. It will bring joy to your soul.

JOY

We all need and deserve joy. What brings one person joy may not to another. The important thing is to find things that bring *you* joy. Being happy is on the surface…feeling good about the external things in your life. Joy comes from *within* you, down in your heart. Do you know the song "Joy, joy, joy, joy down in my heart, down in my heart…"? Joy is what you feel deep inside. That's the difference between being happy and feeling joy.

LAUGHTER

Norman Cousins says "Laughter is the best medicine." I have to agree. It can lower your blood pressure, change your mood, and lift your spirit. Laughter is a must in order to get through life. Laughter helps you cope better and not take life so seriously.

People take life way too seriously. There is enough negativity and stress in the world without adding to it by being tense and angry. I have experienced many frustrating situations, but when I feel down, I do my best to see the positivity or humor. Maybe it comes out as sarcasm, but if it makes you laugh, you're way ahead of the game.

One technique to get yourself to laugh is to imagine the person that upset you in their underwear or naked. Another idea is to imagine that person as a small child. You can also watch a funny movie, read something funny, or think of a particular situation that really cracked you up in the past.

If someone can make you laugh during a tough time, they have given you a gift.

LAUGHING AT YOURSELF

Being able to laugh at yourself can make all the difference in how you handle situations. People who are not able to laugh go through life angry and grumpy and take themselves way too seriously. People who can laugh at themselves tend to be more relaxed, fun and happy.

If you feel you have had a bad day or have messed something up, try to find the humor in it. It will help you see the situation in a different way and not seem so terrible. When you laugh at yourself, you are coping with the stress of the situation and releasing the tension. We know about tension, anger, and frustration. Let it go and laugh.

OBSERVING NATURE

Being in nature is a great way to de-stress, relax, and be in the moment. Nature is soothing but also healing. Nature gives off positive energy. Anytime you are feeling tired, stressed, or drained, try getting out in nature.

Being in nature is relaxing, but observing nature can take you into a whole new world. Many times I have sat on my front porch observing nature. I have seen everything from deer, fox, rabbits, and opossum to insects, spiders, and toads.

One night I sat on my porch in deep thought about something that was bothering me. I saw a toad on my patio and stopped to observe it. The toad ate a beetle, then another and another. The more he ate, the more I was intrigued. I sat and watched this amazing creature eat forty-three bugs in one bug-hunting session! It was amazing to imagine forty-three good-sized beetles inside that tiny stomach!

It may sound like I had no life, at the time, for me to sit and watch that toad, but I came to realize that not only did I learn something, my nature observation had taken my mind off the concerns I had had before spotting the toad. I was in the moment. I also noticed that I was now looking at whatever I had been worrying about in a different way and with less magnitude.

Being in the moment is very therapeutic and helps us to remember that not all that we worry about is as bad as we imagine. So, next time you are stressed or worried about something, take a break from it and get out in nature. See the trees, feel the breeze, watch a bug, or absorb the healing energy. You'll be glad you did. It will relax your mind and heal your soul.

SUNSHINE THERAPY

Sunshine therapy is about relaxing in the sun. The sun is relaxing and healing. The sun helps warm your muscles and relax them. The sun can bless you with vitamin D (this is the best way to obtain it). I am not talking about abusing the sun, just relaxing in it for a minimum of fifteen to twenty minutes per day.

Sunshine therapy helps lift our spirits. We are usually all very happy to see the sun after several days of rain. That's because we need the sun. It helps our bones grow, heals our physical wounds, and relaxes our bodies.

When you get a chance, take a break from work or from life and relax in the sun for that fifteen or twenty minutes. It will do your mind, body and spirit some good. (See Healing Effects of the Sun handout in Appendix)

STRETCHING

Stretching is a great way to release stress. Stretching your muscles is vital for oxygen to get in and help rebuild them, making them better and stronger. Stretching also soothes and relaxes your soul, which makes it a soul activity. (See Stretching section.)

YOGA

Yoga is a great soul activity. Yoga helps us relax, strengthen, and center ourselves. Yoga balances out your body, mind and soul. (See Yoga section.)

MASSAGE

Massage is one of my top five favorite things to do. It relaxes the muscles, eases the mind, and soothes the soul. Not only is massage therapeutic for the body, but it is also a great way to release stress, negativity, and toxins.

Give yourself a gift: get a massage. It is one way to tell your body that you love it and appreciate it. Think about how much your body does for you every day...all of the activities it performs, day in and day out...every day, every year. Appreciate all of the functions it performs, internal and external. Your body is an amazing organism. Appreciate it.

While experiencing a massage, I think "body appreciation." When my feet are being massaged, I appreciate what my feet do for me every day. When my legs are being massaged, I appreciate what my legs do for me every day. And so on. During my massages, I send all body parts total love and appreciation. And, I do my best to be in the moment (who wants to escape the experience of massage)?

Show your body appreciation. Get a massage. Be in the moment. It heals your body and soothes your soul.

Benefits of Massage
*Decreases blood pressure
*Improves immune system
*Increases relaxation
*Helps alleviate headaches
*Decreases pain

*Decreases muscle spasms

*Decreases stress

*Decreases stiffness

*Improves circulation

*Improves range of motion

*Decreases muscle soreness

BODY APPRECIATION

I have been an aerobics instructor for over twelve years and have been exercising for over twenty-three years. I have put a lot of exercise on this body over the years and let me tell you, it's amazing how it's held up. I've eaten very healthy for years, and that helps, but still, this body of mine has taken a pounding. We're talking anywhere from one workout a day for six or seven days a week to three to five workouts per day, five or six days a week, for years. Once, I taught sixteen classes in a week just subbing for other instructors. I was known as the "sub queen." That was too much for my body, I believe. But that was all back when I thought I was indestructible.

There came a time when I experienced pain in both knees. The pain and throbbing was unsettling and stopped me in my tracks. It continued for five or six days straight, really scaring me. During that time, I did a lot of soul searching. I had concerns that I would not be able to exercise again and wondered what I would do for a living.

One day I got out of the shower and started to put lotion on my body the way I normally do, but this time I slowed down and thought. I thought of all the times I had taught this exercise class and that exercise class. I thought of all the times I had subbed for this person and that, this week and that week, this year and that year. I started to regret all the exercise classes I had taught and the times I had subbed for other people's classes. Then I started to cry. I felt as if I had given my knees to all these other people, and was now left with knees that did not work well. I realized that I had identified myself as being only a fitness instructor, as if there were nothing else I could do for a living.

Then I stopped myself. I stopped the negative spiral and started thinking about how much I had given to students, how I had motivated them and helped them be healthy. I thought of the times I had subbed a class for an instructor whose dad was in the hospital, or the one who wanted to take her mother for lunch on Mother's Day, or the one who had to go to a funeral. I began to realize that this body of mine had helped a lot of people do a lot of things that they might not otherwise have been able to do. I realized that even though I had over-exercised through the years, I had given of myself and my body to help others. I cried, feeling appreciation for my body and my knees. I rubbed the lotion on my legs and felt deep appreciation for what my body was and what it had given others. Then, I appreciated the fact that my body and knees had also given *me* good health by exercising all those years.

After that day, I would put lotion on as before, but being *in the moment* and having total appreciation for my body. I appreciated my toes for balance, my ankles and legs for walking, running, and jumping. I appreciated my core, abs, chest, back, arms, hands, fingers, and neck. I sent love to every body part while putting lotion on each particular part.

A week passed, and my knees healed. They have been great ever since. However, I do not pound my body into the ground like I used to. Now, I respect it, listen to it, and appreciate it. If it speaks to me, I listen. As I tell my class participants, personal training and nutrition clients, "Listen to your body. In the beginning, your body whispers to you. If you don't listen to it, it will talk to you. If you don't listen, it will yell at you. If you don't listen, it will scream at you. If you don't listen, it will cry." Listen to your body. Respect it. Appreciate it. You'll be glad you did.

REAL SPIRITUALITY

Where do I begin with this subject? I can write something that makes some people happy, most people happy, or I can just write what I believe and you can take from it what you want.

Spirituality is, I believe, the biggest "soul activity" there is. Believing in a higher power can help strengthen you, balance you, or soothe your soul. Spirituality gives us something to believe in, but more importantly, it helps us cope with everyday life. We all know not every day is perfect. Some days can be challenging. But believing in God, the Universe, or a higher power can reduce stress, comfort you, and heal your soul.

I was raised as a Methodist and went to church, Bible school, confirmation, the whole nine yards. After becoming an adult, I turned away from church due to a judgmental experience I had as a high-schooler. I felt as if I had been judged unfairly by a couple I had just met. Something did not sit well with me after that day, especially since it had occurred in the church.

Soon I was in college and never "had" to go to church. It was one of those sweet freedoms I experienced at college. No parents around to tell me what to do or how to do it. I continued this freedom for years until I got married and had a daughter. All of a sudden I felt this urge to take my daughter to church. To this day, I don't think she remembers church, since she was only ten months old at the time. Maybe it was a calling for *me* to go back to church and I just *thought* it was for my daughter.

I said a few prayers asking God to help me find a church without having to "church hop." Within days, I spoke to a lady about a new church that she went to. I never brought it up in conversation; *she did.* Come to find out, the church was being held in an elementary school directly across the street from the new house we had just moved into! I thought that was quite a coincidence. I was told that the church was nondenominational and that, for me, took the pressure off. It was definitely convenient, so I went. I dropped my daughter off at the nursery and went to the service by myself, not knowing a soul there. The service was in the school gymnasium, the choir was in regular clothes, and the pastor wore khakis and a shirt.

As the choir started to sing, I felt something. Whatever it was, it brought me to tears. It was a bit embarrassing to be crying in front of a bunch of strangers before the service had even started, but I could not contain it. It was an energy that surrounded me and brought up emotion from who knows where. For the first time, I actually felt what I call "the presence of God."

After that, I loved going to church and went every Sunday. It made me feel good, accepted, and relaxed. I could wear shorts and flip-flops to church if I wanted to! This was not what I was used to. Growing up, we had to wear a dress or something "real nice."

Everything was great for about two years, until this one particular sermon I went to. The pastor, all of a sudden, started talking about sinning and sinners. Hearing those words made me feel uncomfortable. Later, for some reason, I felt guilt, and not sure what I had done to feel the guilt. I stopped going to church.

I moved to Atlanta and got into hiking. Hiking became my heaven. Hiking and nature soon became my new "church." I felt closer to God out in nature than I ever did in church. Now, I am not saying that God isn't in church. I believe he is everywhere. What I *am* saying is that hiking and nature was *my* way of creating my own spirituality. I believe you should do whatever works for you. Some people like to worship in church with others, some like to meditate and communicate with God alone. I just happened to like communicating in nature.

There are many ways to develop your own spirituality. It may be in organized religion, nature, meditation, or it may be singing and listening to spiritual music. Some people like to watch church services on TV.

For many years I read spiritual books, and still do. Reading many different spiritual books helped me find my way down this new road of spirituality. I read a variety of books that helped me discover different viewpoints. It was a process that helped me realize what my thoughts, feelings, and beliefs were. The most impactful spiritual books for me were the *Conversations with God* series by Neale Donald Walsch. I have read them and re-read them, and obtained the CDs as well.

Whatever your spirituality, it doesn't matter, as long as it's the right fit for you. You are the one who needs to be comfortable with it. Spirituality can be a very personal thing. It can be private, or it can be social. What's important is that you find something that works for you—something that makes you feel good and helps you learn, grow, and cope with life.

I am a strong believer that spirituality can reduce stress and lift you up. Whatever road you take, know that spirituality can be an incredible soul activity.

BELIEF IN GOD VS. RELATIONSHIP WITH GOD

Believing in God is simply believing that He (or a higher power) exists. Having a relationship with God is what it sounds like: a relationship. Being in a relationship with God, I believe, is when you talk to God on a regular basis. You talk, God listens, then God talks and you listen. You are talking to God like you would your best friend, only better. I don't see it as formal prayer all the time, but a conversation in which you feel comfortable saying anything at any time and where God loves and accepts you no matter what.

I "believed" in God for years as I was growing up. It's what I was taught. I wasn't sure what God was, really, but I was told that there was a God. We went to church to worship this man/thing/being called God. Now we couldn't see him, but I was told he was there, in church and everywhere. How do you believe in something that you cannot see? As a child, I believed my parents because parents are adults, and adults know much more than children…right?

Well, I went along with this "God thing" because I was told it was so. Around age fourteen, I thought I would test this guy named God. My first "boyfriend" from middle school had given me a ring with a blue stone in it. Well, somehow I lost it. I remember looking all over the place for this new ring (from a BOY!). I thought I had looked everywhere. After searching high and low, I said a prayer to this guy named God. I prayed, and prayed, and prayed, asking him to help me find the ring I'd lost. Sure enough, within a few minutes, I found it… underneath the couch. I could have sworn that I had already looked there, but it didn't matter because I found it. I thanked God so much for helping me out that day and I never forgot it.

I know I was only fourteen years old, but this made an impact on me. It was the first time I thought that maybe all these people were right. Maybe there was, indeed, a God. I was in a bind that day, he helped me out after I asked for his help, and I never forgot it. It was the first time I remember talking or praying to God on my own, outside of church. I believed there was a God because of my *own* experience, not based on *what others said*.

As I grew up, I continued to believe, but it wasn't until age twenty-nine or thirty that I started delving into spirituality. I read *Embraced by the Light* by Betty Eadie. It wowed me. I thought it was great! It had all the answers you ever wanted to know about heaven, angels, and so on. Where had this book been all this time? Did people know about this? I was so engrossed in the book and the questions it answered. Little did I know then that I was beginning my spiritual journey.

After that book, I read angel book after angel book. I couldn't seem to get enough of them. Until one day I got to a point where I felt I had read every angel story out there and moved on to James Redfield's *The Celestine Prophecy*. I didn't normally read fiction, but people kept saying how good it was. It was. It was different, but good…I guess. I don't think I truly understood that book until years later. But I was on my spiritual journey and loving it.

I grew spiritually for years, but grew so much more after moving to Austin. The city of Austin introduced me to a friend who then introduced me to a self-growth training in Dallas. I had always been into self-improvement, but I had reached a point in my life where I felt stuck—as if I didn't fit into my own life anymore. It was as if I were ready for something different, on a different level. So I signed up for all three personal growth trainings.

The night I secured my registration with my credit card, I had the strangest experience. It was like no other. Some would call it a dream, but this was like no dream I'd ever had. I was in nature and flying high above the trees, yet able to see every detail of them far below me. Then there was suddenly white all around me. I felt light, free, and happy, but wondering why I was floating in all white. Then I heard a voice. It was not a man's voice, nor a woman's. It was an asexual voice. It said, "I am hungry for you." That was it. I woke up in my bed and thought, "Oh, I am back inside my body"…then, "Oh, I am back in my bed." Then, "Oh, I am back in my bedroom," then, "Oh, I am back in my apartment." It was as if I had had an out of body experience. This may not sound strange to you...but the strange part came *after* I became oriented.

I was lying in my bed, wide awake, and tears were coming down my face. The tears were continuous, but I was not crying. I was not emotional, I was not upset; I was not even experiencing the irregular breathing that a person does when crying. I felt perfectly fine emotionally, except that tears kept running down my face, nonstop. And my nose was stuffed up as if I were crying...but I was not crying. I was not crying in the "dream," and I was not crying or upset when I returned to consciousness. I felt a little bewildered, wondering what had just happened, but I was perfectly fine emotionally. I could not understand how and why the tears were streaming down my face without feeling the emotion. They wouldn't stop...I was so freaked out by this experience that I decided to journal it, or at least write it down so I would not forget it once I went back to sleep.

As I wrote, the tears continued to fall, even though I felt fine. When I stopped writing to think, the tears stopped. When I started writing again, the tears started again. When I stopped writing, they stopped. This went on for fifteen or twenty minutes. I was so perplexed by it all. Once I finished writing about the "dream" and the experience afterwards, the tears stopped and my nose cleared up immediately. This was the strangest thing that had ever happened to me. I could not explain it. It did not make any sense.

At 1:30 a.m., I called the friend who had told me about the training I had signed up for the night before. I told her about the experience and how strange it was. As I was explaining my experience, I started to cry, this time with emotion. The next day, I told my mother, and again, as I explained my experience to her, I cried with emotion. The experience was not scary or upsetting, but for some reason, emotion came up whenever I told someone about it.

My question is, why did the emotion come up when telling people about the experience, but not while it happened? Why were all those tears coming down involuntarily for those fifteen or twenty minutes, with no internal emotion? Why did they stop when I stopped writing and start again when I started writing?

Strange experience…

The way I make sense of it is this: I believe my soul was the voice I heard telling me it was hungry for me. I believe it knew what I was ready to embark upon…huge steps in self-growth. I did not know at the time what I was in for with the trainings. Looking back, they were a huge leap forward in self-growth, emotional cleansing, and spirituality, even though the trainings were very neutral and non-religion based.

CLOSER TO GOD

My next huge spiritual leap was after the death of my mother. By this time I already had a solid relationship with God. Little did I know how much more I was to grow. My mother's passing was the most devastating thing I had ever experienced. The pain, anger, frustration, confusion, and depression were enough to almost destroy me.

I had not experienced pain like this ever before. It was the most excruciating emotional pain I have ever experienced. The best way I can explain it is to call it gut-wrenching. Each time I cried (which was often), it felt as if someone were putting a shovel in my gut and jumping on it with all their weight, over and over again.

Although the experience was devastating and gut-wrenching, it deepened my relationship with God and brought me closer to him. Now, I am not saying that I threw my hands up in the air and said, "Ok, that's fine, my mother died." No, I yelled and kicked and screamed. I was angry, and cried about her being gone, about me being without her, and at God for taking her. Deep down, I knew she was in a better place and that she was out of pain. I knew it was best. But it still didn't make my pain go away. My mind could handle it intellectually, but my heart bled.

Time helps, yes: a lot of it. But does the pain ever really go away? Whatever the answer, it was a done deal and I couldn't change things. The good that came out of the pain were the steps I took closer to God. Now, when I am upset or in pain, I turn to God. I talk to him *much* more than before, and I listen. I also turn on spiritual music and it helps heal my heart. Before, I would just feel low and sometimes pray about my situation, but now I immediately turn to God, Jesus, angels, guides, Archangel Michael, and my mother for comfort when the pain becomes too much.

And you know what? It works every time. I can cry and cry, but after talking it out with God, Jesus, angels, guides, Archangel Michael, and my Mom, the pain dissipates and I feel a sense of peace come over me. It's amazing how it works. It can be the most painful, gut-wrenching cry, but in an instant it's gone and replaced with the most beautiful peace.

CHOOSING GOD

Another situation that drew me closer to God was the end of a toxic relationship. This relationship was good, bad, up, down, beautiful, and ugly...often. I reached a point where I felt I was going crazy. I didn't feel that way every day, but I did feel it often. I kept asking myself what was wrong. What was I doing wrong? Why was this happening? I had worked on myself emotionally and spiritually—and I mean hard—for the previous seven years. Why was this not working?

I would ask myself and God, where's the joy? The laughter? The lightness and freedom to be who I am and be loved and accepted? It wasn't that I wasn't doing the work. I worked very hard on myself. I believed that if I worked hard enough on myself, then things would work out beautifully—that I would be rewarded with this incredibly healthy, loving, committed, and fulfilling relationship.

Not to say there weren't good times and some fun...but only 20 percent of the time? That's just not right. I understand that we all go through tough times and stick it out, are supportive to others and get supported...that it makes us stronger and better, that it makes the relationship stronger. I get all that. But to have only 20 percent of the relationship be happy? Something's not right.

After many draining, exhausting arguments and discussions, I learned two very important things. First, you can work as hard as you want on yourself and the relationship, but if the other person does not, the relationship is stuck in the mud. I know sometimes that you have to go through the mud to get to the meadow, but if you are constantly stuck in the mud, you need to learn how to get out. You can work and work and work at it, but if you're stuck, you may need help getting out. It takes two people—and God—to make a relationship work. If the other person is willing to clean up his or her dirt and you are willing to clean up yours, then you can have a dirt-free relationship. If one person is not willing to clean up their dirt, then you just get dirty all over again, time and time again.

Now, you can both help one another clean each other's dirt...to a point. At some point, each person is going to have to do his or her own cleaning. I can't expect anyone else to rid me of my pain over the loss of my mother. Others can try their best to comfort and soothe my pain, but ultimately, I am the one who needs to go through the grieving process. I am the one who needs to find (hopefully) healthy ways to express my pain and to release it until my heart heals.

The other person, at some point too, needs to heal their own emotional wounds. Others can be comforted to a point, but ultimately, they have to heal their own wounds. The healing process goes much more quickly if someone is proactive in the healing process. Someone may have the tools to help him- or herself, but if not, healing may take longer.

The other consideration is that each person has to be willing to heal or want to heal. Some people have a need to stay in pain longer than others or are not aware they are stuck. I believe the saying, "*You can lead a horse to water, but you cannot make him drink.*" The horse will drink when it's thirsty. So, no matter how much you want to help someone, they have to be willing. Overall, we are all responsible for cleaning our own dirt, or healing our own pain.

The second thing I learned through all of the relationship toxicity is to choose God first. I had been married and divorced, twice. I had had enough relationships to know when they were not working. They weren't fulfilling. I was repeating a pattern and the pattern was getting old.

One night, I got into a toxic argument in my toxic relationship. I got so upset that I felt as if I were going to "lose it"…but I didn't. Actually, the toxic argument pushed me into choosing God over anyone else. At that point, I expressed my choice and was not going to budge. I came to realize that God's love was *so* much more fulfilling and comforting than anything I had experienced in the past. So, duh, why not choose God over anyone else? I had never done that in the past. I had never told any man, "I choose God over you." I had never told God, "I choose you over anyone else." But I did that night. The guy left out of frustration and rejection. After that, I told God again, "I choose you. If I am to be alone, then fine. I still choose you."

And you know what? An inner peace came over me. I felt loved, full of clarity, and very confident in my choice. All of a sudden, the heavy weight was gone, and the angst, the frustration, and everything negative that went along with it. The heaviness was replaced with a beautiful inner peace. I felt loved, full of clarity, and very confident in my choice. It felt that everything was going to be just fine. I felt it and I believed it.

I will never forget that night. As I thought about it, it became clear to me. That's why I had not had fulfilling relationships in the past. They all had one thing in common. No spirituality. No connection with God. No partner that was connected to God or who had a real relationship with God…and not being partners with God. God was the missing link in my past relationships. This time, I got it…I really got it about God and relationships.

Because of my much deeper relationship with God, I turn to him always for the good and the not so good. And you know what? He is always there…I mean, *always* there. He supports me. He lifts me up when I am down, and catches me when I fall. He comforts me when I am angry, hurt, frustrated, or confused. He is with me always in one way or another. He may be in an answer to a prayer, the words in a song, a movie I see, a book I read, or a person I meet. No matter where I go or where I turn, God is there. Just as I learned as a little girl, God is not just in church; He is everywhere.

GRATITUDE

Gratitude is about being grateful for anything and everything in your life. Gratitude is the appreciation of having a job, a roof over your head, wonderful friends and family in your life, having the eyes to see scenic nature, ears to hear beautiful music, taste buds to savor delicious foods, and the incredible feeling of touch.

A great way to shift yourself out of a bad mood is to think—or better yet, write—about the blessings you have been given in your life. Pick up a pen and write down at least five things that you are grateful for. It is a good way to pull yourself out of the "poor me" syndrome. There are so many things to be grateful for. The list is endless.

You will see that what you thought was a bad day is not so bad if you think about how things could be worse. For example, let's say your boss reprimands you or doesn't appreciate the fact that you put in extra hours on a particular project. Think about the many people in the world who don't have a job. Or you may complain about wanting a bigger house, only to remember that many people do not have a home. You may complain that your body is overweight or doesn't look the way you'd like it to, only to be reminded that some people have no food, or even no legs to walk with.

It's all about remembering what you have and knowing that there are many others out there who have so much less. However, less can be more. The less people have, the more they seem to appreciate what they do have. Whatever you are unhappy with or are complaining about can always be taken away. When you think of it that way, it makes you appreciate what you *do* have. That's the key to gratitude: focus on what you *do* have, not on what you don't have.

Let's be **real** here. We're going to get down from time to time. When I lived in Dallas, I applied for a particular job in advertising. I interviewed for it and wanted it with all my heart. I called to follow up, only to find that the job had been given to someone else. I was very disappointed and upset. I got in my car and drove to a quiet place to cry. After crying about the situation, I thought: this does not feel good…what could make me feel better? I decided to pull out a pen and write down all of the things that I was grateful for. The list was much longer than I had expected and you know what? I felt so much better after making the list. Ok, that's easy when it's something minor. What about when it is a real difficult or painful situation?

The loss of my mother was difficult. Sure, it was painful, but I still found positive things in the situation. I thought about the fact that she was no longer in pain. I thought about the forty-five years of love and wonderful experiences that *I did* have. Some people do not have a mother at all growing up. I was blessed to have an incredible mother. I was grateful for having her in my life for all those years.

Another blessing that came from this painful situation was being able to relate to those who have lost their mother or other loved one. The experience helped me to understand and create a bond with these people. It will also help me comfort those in the future when a loved one is lost.

There are always things to be grateful for. We just need to remember what they are. Remembering what we are blessed with helps us to practice gratitude. So, when things get tough, remember the saying, "Have an attitude of gratitude." You'll live a richer, fuller life and feel much better.

YOUR LIFE'S PURPOSE

There comes a time in your life where you wonder why you are here. Why were we put here on earth? What are we supposed to do while we are here?

Sure, we can all go through the motions unconsciously and live an average life. Or we can live consciously and live a life that is purposeful.

There was a time when my life was going pretty well. Everything seemed just fine, but something was missing. I wasn't sure what it was, but there was a void. I didn't want a big house, a Mercedes, a swimming pool or a boat; I'd had those in the past. What I missed was something that was not materialistic; it was internal. This need for purpose, to feel fulfilled, was hard to explain. I knew that I had to do something worthwhile on this earth—something that would make a difference in people's lives. I wanted to make a positive impact through health, fitness, nutrition, spirituality, healing, and wellness.

There came a time when I didn't feel I could go about my life without taking action on these feelings. Then I met a woman who recommended a book to me. It was my first time meeting her and out of nowhere, she blurted out its title and recommended that I read it. I never saw her again.

Funny how things happen at the "right" time. Here I was, wanting to move forward in finding or fulfilling my purpose! The book this woman recommended was *The Life You Were Born to Live: A Guide to Finding Your Life Purpose*, by Dan Millman. She wrote it down for me and that was it.

I kept the paper she wrote on for several weeks. Every few days the book title would pop into my mind. I've learned over the years that when something keeps coming back to me, it's usually trying to tell me something. So I ordered the book and read it.

Maybe you already know what you want to do. If you do, go for it. If you don't, try the book I mentioned, or just pay attention. Pay attention to your thoughts, your talents, skills, knowledge, and experience. Most of all, pay attention to what you are passionate about. If you have a passion for something, you will do it well. Listen to that inner voice. You'll know it…the one that never really goes away. The voice or dream that keeps creeping back into your mind is just a reminder that it still wants to be created.

LISTENING TO YOUR INNER VOICE

Listening to your inner voice is about listening to your soul. It's the most important guide you can ever listen to. Think about it…there are so many voices we listen to, day in and day out, year after year. There are the unknown voices on the television and radio. There are the known voices like our friends, families, mothers, fathers, siblings, spouses, bosses, relatives, children, and significant others. We are listening to voices all day long, every day. These voices are telling us what we should do or not do with our lives, our jobs, our marriages, our families and our health.

It's no wonder that we are all stressed. So many voices, yet so little space to hear it all.

Then there is the question of *whom* to listen to. Which voices have the *most* to say, the *most important* thing to say, or the *right* thing to say?

The next question is, "Which voice knows the right thing to do for *your* life? Which voice has *your* best interests in mind? Or does it have *its own* best interests in mind?

That's the key word…in *mind*. It doesn't matter what voice you listen to, or what interest it has in mind. Staying in our minds can drive us crazy. Getting out of our minds and into our souls is where our best interests lie. Going deep within ourselves is the place we need to go and listen. That's why getting away from it all can be such a great thing. You leave behind all the confusing voices, and can actually *hear*.

There is a picture I have of a boat on a peaceful lake. At the bottom, there is a quote that says, *"The quieter you become, the more you can hear."* It's so true. Once we disconnect from the voices in the world, we can listen to our own inner voice: the voice that knows us and knows what's best for us. Our inner voice knows what we need to do and what we need not do. Our inner voice can sometimes be hard to hear if we don't become quiet. No matter how loud life becomes, our inner voice is always there, speaking to us, whispering to us. It never goes away.

Your inner voice has all the answers, right there inside of you. So why do we go looking for answers from others? Do we think that others know us better than we know ourselves? Or know our lives better than we know them?

You are the one who knows you best. You know what is best for you and your life. Just listen. If you can't hear it, get quiet. It's there, waiting to be heard.

TRUSTING YOUR INNER VOICE

Once you listen to your inner voice, the next step is to trust it. Listening to your inner voice and trusting it can be different things.

Learning to trust your inner voice can be difficult if you don't trust yourself. Learning to trust yourself is knowing what's best for you. Remember that you are you. No one else is you, or knows you better than you do. Who else is better to trust with you and your life than you?

If you have a problem trusting your inner voice, do things to improve your self-esteem. Write or say positive affirmations, speak up for yourself, value and honor your feelings. Remind yourself that you know yourself better than anyone else. This is *your* life, and *you* know what's best for you.

ACTING ON YOUR INNER VOICE

Once you listen to your inner voice and trust it, you need to act on it. Acting on your inner voice can be the toughest part. There may be times when acting on your inner voice will be easy, and times when it will go against all else. This is when most people, do not act on their inner voice: when it goes against what their friends and family say, or what their co-workers do, and so on. There may be times when everyone else thinks you are weird or crazy, but your *true* inner voice is not weird or crazy.

There have been times when I needed to let go of certain jobs, people, beliefs, or behaviors for one reason or another. Maybe they were unhealthy, or maybe I just outgrew them. At times like these I may have felt guilt, frustration, or sadness, but knew deep down what I needed to do. Taking the step of acting on your inner voice may be challenging, but once you do it, you'll feel surprisingly lighter. You'll feel a sense of relief—as if you've lost fifty pounds (or more)!

Just know that there are three steps regarding your inner voice: *Listen. Trust. Act.* Once you complete all three, your life will change for the better. Remember, it's easy to go along with the crowd, but it is *empowering* to follow your soul. If you listen, trust, and act on what your soul tells you, you may not be like everyone else, but I guarantee that you'll be happy about who you are and what you are becoming.

REAL YOU

REALNESS VS PERFECTIONISM

Realness comes from acting on your inner voice.

Perfectionism comes from fear…

Fear of not being good enough…

Fear of being judged by others.

Let it go.

You ARE good enough. Now. Today. Every day.

If you don't believe it,

Think it.

Say it.

Write it…10 times every day.

You will come to believe it.

Note: If you found any errors while reading this book, it's okay. I left them there intentionally—as a reminder to let go of perfectonsm. And to replace it with Realness.

☺

Conclusion

Real health is not just one thing. It is a combination of many things. It's difficult to be perfectly healthy in all areas, but who's perfect? No one, right? So do your best in each category for your own health and wellness and see where it takes you. Wellness is not something that happens overnight. It takes time, energy, education, and experience to know what works for you and your life. Everyone lives life differently, but we all have the same basic needs.

The road to wellness is:
*Real Food
*Real Exercise (strength training, cardio, flexibility, and balance)
*Real Water, Air, and Cleansing
*Real Weight, Metabolism, and Hormones
*Real Rest and Physical Healing
*Real Nature and Sunshine
*Real Emotional Health and Healing
*Real Positive Attitude and Environment
*Real Soul Activities and Spirituality

I've tried to provide these here: basic needs and options for you to choose from to fulfill those needs. Remember, it's *your* body and *your* life. Do what you can for you. Do what you can live with. Most of all, please don't be too hard on yourself. Things happen. Some you control, and some you don't.

Overall...
Love,
Honor,
And Value Yourself,
by being your own best friend.
In the end, **that** is what *Real Health, Real Life* is all about.

In health, healing and realness,

Jillian Lambert

SUMMARY (reproduced as a handout in Appendix)

Wellness Lifestyle Goals Worksheet

Body Composition: Lean tissue vs. fat tissue

GOAL:

Flexibility: Complete range of motion. Stretch all major muscle groups after exercise. Hold each stretch for ten seconds or more. This allows the oxygen to get into the muscle. The oxygen helps to rebuild the muscle stronger and better.

Recommendation: five to twenty minutes once per day, hold each stretch for ten seconds or longer.

GOAL:

Cardiovascular: Running, walking, hiking, swimming, aerobics, kickboxing, cycling, rebounding, etc. Fat starts to burn after the fifteen- to twenty-minute mark of exercise. (Your body burns glycogen until then.) Twenty to sixty minutes, four or five times per week

GOAL:

Strength Training: Weight machines, free weights, stability ball, resistance bands, etc. These activities strengthen all of the major muscle groups. two or three times per week every other day, or alternate muscle groups every other day. Muscles need forty-eight hours of rest after you work them.

GOAL:

Balance: Stability and coordination. Tools to improve balance are stability ball, Bosu, wobbleboard, and coreboard. Yoga also helps improve balance.

GOAL:

Soul Activities/Relaxation: Yoga, tai chi, meditation, reading, spirituality, art, massage, time in nature, bubble baths, hobbies, and so on.

GOAL:

Nutrition: Eat *lots* of raw fruits and vegetables. Eat healthy proteins, carbs, and fats.

Lean protein includes fish, tofu, chicken, and lean cuts of beef.

Healthy carbs: fruit, sprouted grain bread.

Healthy fats: avocados, coconut oil, flax seed oil, olive oil.

GOAL:

Water: Take your weight in pounds and divide in half. This is how many ounces you should drink daily. (For example, someone who weighs 120 lbs. should drink 60 ounces of water per day.)

GOAL:

Rest: Getting enough sleep keeps your fat burning process running efficiently. Lack of sleep slows the fat burning process. Get seven to nine hours of continuous sleep each night if possible.

GOAL:

Sunshine: The sun can help lift your mood, heal wounds, help with some forms of acne and eczema, and is also the best form of vitamin D. Get fifteen to twenty minutes of early morning sunshine each day.

GOAL:

Nature: Nature calms and heals us. Get out in nature at least once or twice a week—more often if possible. Time alone to think is very beneficial to your mental state and your physical wellbeing. This quiet time can be used to sort out problems, create new ideas, or just relax.

GOAL:

Positivity: A positive attitude makes a big difference in how you cope with life. Look on the bright side and see the good in things. Positive thinking is a great boost for your health. See positive. Think positive. Speak positive. Be positive.

FREQUENTLY ASKED QUESTIONS

Q. What is holistic health?

A. Holistic health is about keeping the *whole* body healthy in a natural way, and without drugs or surgery. Whole body health approaches health through mind, body, and spirit.

Q. What is the most effective and efficient exercise for the lower body?

A. The most effective exercises for the lower body are lunges. Lunges work many large muscles, including quadriceps (front thigh), gluteus maximus (butt), hamstrings (back of thighs), and gastrocnemius (calves). Lunges also work the stabilizing muscles: abs, back, and inner and outer thighs.

Types of lunges can include forward, reverse, stationary, and walking. They are all effective for different reasons. Forward lunges work the front of the legs more, while reverse lunges work the back of the legs and are easier on the knees. Stationary lunges improve balance, working the stabilizing muscles. Walking lunges are the most challenging and, I believe, are the most effective.

Q. What is the most effective and efficient exercise for the upper body?

A. The most effective exercise for the upper body is pushups. Yes, everybody loves pushups. The reason most people are not fond of pushups is because they are challenging. But they are very effective. Pushups work the pectoralis major (chest), anterior deltoid (front shoulder), and triceps (upper back of arm) all at the same time. You can make pushups more interesting by doing them on your toes, knees, stability ball, bench, a step, or up against the wall.

Q. What is the healthiest way to eat?

A. The healthiest way to eat is fruits, vegetables, and proteins. Fruits and vegetables should be raw. Proteins should be lean. In addition to fish chicken and turkey, nuts and seeds are also a great source of protein. Make sure nuts and seeds are *raw*, not cooked, oiled, or roasted. (If you include grains, make sure you go with whole grains. Sprouted grain bread, like Ezekiel Bread, is one of the healthiest.)

Q. What are the best fruits to eat?

A. All fruits are great. Raw fruits are best. The larger the variety of fruits you eat, the better. Eat the "Rainbow Way," which means to include foods of a wide range of different colors.

Q. What are the best vegetables to eat?

A. Vegetables are healthiest when eaten raw. Raw vegetables have "live" enzymes that enhance your health. Cooking vegetables destroys the enzymes. The larger variety of vegetables you eat, the better. Eat the "Rainbow Way," which means to include foods of a wide range of different colors.

FREQUENTLY ASKED QUESTIONS

Q. What is Real Health?
A. Real Health consists of nine important factors:

1. **Real Food** (raw, organic, whole foods)
2. **Real Exercise** (physical and mental)
3. **Real Water and Air** (clean, pure, filtered water and air)
4. **Real Weight and Metabolism** (maintaining your Real Body Weight)
5. **Real Rest** (quality sleep)
6. **Real Nature** (getting in touch with nature one or two times a week. Every day is best)
7. **Real Sunshine** (fifteen to twenty minutes of early morning sun daily.)
8. **Real Relaxation / Spirituality** (music, painting, massage, hot bath, meditation prayer)
9. **Real Love / Positive Attitude / Emotional Health** (healthy relationships with self and others, positive thinking, affirmations, motivation, self-help books, journaling, counseling and self-love)

Q. How do I speed up my metabolism?
A. Metabolism can be affected by food, exercise, alcohol, sleep, hormones and of course, genetics. Foods that can help increase your metabolism are high in fiber, protein, or calcium. Exercise can speed up your metabolism through weight lifting and interval training. Staying away from alcohol and getting enough quality sleep can improve your body's fat burning process. Genetics? Be born with "skinny genes!"

Q. Why is sunshine considered healthy?
A. Getting enough sunshine helps the body create vitamin D, which is important for strong, healthy bones and teeth. Sunshine is the best form of vitamin D. Sunshine also lifts your mood, heals bones, injuries,

217

and skin disorders. Early morning sunshine exposure of fifteen to twenty minutes a day is best (daily if possible). Early morning sunshine *without* sunscreen is best because sunscreen stops the sun from producing vitamin D in the skin.

JILLIAN'S HEALTH
ROUTINE

6:30 a.m.   Rife machine detox: 33 min.

7:00 a.m.   Drink 12–16 oz. of water (optional: fresh lemon squeezed into water to cleanse liver)

7:00 a.m.   Rebounder, treadmill, weights, dance, yoga, Serenity Stretch or hike for 30–45 min. (Alternate activity each day.) Use upbeat music to get pumped up for the day

7:30 a.m.   Shower/get ready for work, etc.

8:30 a.m.–12 noon Fruit (fresh, preferably organic) or fresh juice until noon

Noon   Lean protein with (preferably raw, organic) vegetable(s), or raw veggie sandwich

2:00–4:00 p.m.   1 qt. Silk unsweetened soy milk

5:00 or 6:00 p.m.   Lean protein with (preferably raw, organic) vegetable

7:30 p.m.   Ionic foot bath one or two times per week

9:30 or 10:00 p.m. Bed (optional Rife machine for whatever feels necessary)

Lavender essential oil for relaxation/sleep

PRODUCTS AUTHOR USES

FOOD

    Fruits (organic if possible)

    Vegetables (organic if possible)

    Lean meats (turkey/chicken; organic if possible)

    Fish (salmon, tuna, and sometimes other fish, but mostly salmon)

    Soy milk (Silk unsweetened, green box)

    Eggs (free-range)

    Raw cheese (organic, raw sharp cheddar) in small amounts

    Purified water every morning upon rising: one 12–16 oz. bottle (optional: fresh lemon juice in water to cleanse the liver)

    Occassionally a Boca Burger (soy burger) and ketchup (on rare occasions)

    Edamame (soy beans)

SUPPLEMENTS

    from VP Nutrition (info@vpnutrition.com 877-335-1509):

    Life Max B (B-complex)

    Life Coral (Calcium/Magnesium)

    LifeZyme (Digestive support)

Life Greens

Quality multi-vitamin (not heated over 118 degrees Fahrenheit during production of product-some companies keep heat between 90-100 degrees Fahrenheit)

Organic Coconut Oil (unrefined)

SKIN CARE

from Free Life (http://freelife.com):

Organic Essentials Facial Cleanser or Energizing Purifying Gel

Organic Essentials Rich Moisturizing Cream

Organic Essentials Facial Scrub

Organic Essentials Replenishing Body Lotion

Another Line of products I sometimes use:

100% Pure Cucumber Juice Cleanser

100% Pure Facial Cleanser

100% Pure Brightening Scrub and Mask

100% Pure Acai Berry Antioxidant Face Cream

Organic, extra, extra virgin olive oil (moisturizer)

Avocado oil (moisturizer)

Organic Coconut Oil (unrefined)

WORKOUT EQUIPMENT

Stability Ball, 55 cm or 65 cm (65 cm balls are for people 5'7" or taller)

Rebounder (mini-trampoline)

Bosu (dome-shaped ½ ball)

Treadmill for interval training

Free weights: 5–30 lbs.

Yoga mat

Nature or Hiking Trail

FORMS OF EXERCISE

Hiking: 1–2 times per week

Yoga: 2–3 times per week

Serenity Stretch: 2–3 times per week

Rebounding: 3–4 times per week

Running (trail running or treadmill): once per week

Interval Training (treadmill): once per week

Core Training: 2–3 times per week

Free Weights/Weight Machines: 2–4 times per week

Cross-Training: once per week

Resistance Training/Stability Ball exercises: 1-2 times per week

Dancing (freeform, swing, two-stepping or soul dancing): 1–2 times per week

HOLISTC HEALTH MACHINES AND/OR PRODUCTS

Rife machine: 4–5 times per week

Ionic foot bath: varies

RECOMMENDED
SELF-HELP BOOKS

RELATIONSHIPS

Dr. Henry Cloud and Dr. John Townsend: *Boundaries*

Brenda Davies, MD: *The 7 Healing Chakras*

Barbara DeAngelis, PhD: *How to Make Love All the Time*

Louise L. Hay: *Love Yourself, Heal Your Life Workbook*

Drs. Kathlyn and Gay Hendricks: *Attracting Genuine Love*

Pia Mellody: *Facing Codependence*

Don Miguel Ruiz: *The Four Agreements* and *The Mastery of Love*

SELF EMPOWERMENT/EMOTIONAL HEALTH/ JOURNALING

Rosemary Althea: *You Own the Power*

Brenda Davies, MD: *The 7 Healing Chakras*

Lynn Grabhorn: *Excuse Me, Your Life is Waiting*

Louise L. Hay: *Love Yourself, Heal Your Life Workbook*

Chris Irwin and Bob Weber: *Horses Don't Lie*

Philipp Keel: *All About Me*

Harriet Lerner, PhD: *The Dance of Anger*

Regena Thomashauer: *Mama Gena's School of Womanly Arts*

LIFE MANAGEMENT
Don Miguel Ruiz: *The Four Agreements*
Richard Carlson, PhD: *Don't Sweat the Small Stuff...and it's all small stuff*
Chérie Carter-Scott: *If Life Is a Game, These Are the Rules*
Shakti Gawain: *Creative Visualization*
Regena Thomashauer: *Mama Gena's School of Womanly Arts*
Brenda Davies, MD: *The 7 Healing Chakras*

SPIRITUAL/PURPOSE/AWARENESS
Sylvia Browne: *Soul's Perfection*
Deepak Chopra: *The Seven Spiritual Laws of Success*
Brenda Davies, MD: *The 7 Healing Chakras*
Betty J. Eadie: *Embraced By the Light*
Bishop E. Bernard Jordan: *The Laws of Thinking*
Dan Millman: *The Life You were Born to Live* and *Way of the Peaceful Warrior*
Eckhart Tolle: *The Power of Now* and *A New Earth*
Neale Donald Walsch: *Conversations With God* (Books 1, 2, and 3)

MOTIVATION/AFFIRMATIONS
Bishop E. Bernard Jordan: *The Laws of Thinking*
Louise L. Hay: *I Can Do It*

BODY/HEALTH/NATURE
Ted Andrews: *Animal-Speak*
Louise L. Hay: *You Can Heal Your Life and Heal Your Body*
Richard Hobday: *The Healing Sun*
Chris Irwin and Bob Weber: *Horses Don't Lie*

Kevin Trudeau: *Natural Cures "They" Don't Want You to Know About*

NUTRITION/HEALTH
Dr. Susan E. Brown, Larry Trivieri, Jr.: *The Acid Alkaline Food Guide*
Harvey and Marilyn Diamond: *Fit for Life*
Dr. Douglas N. Graham: *Grain Damage* and *Nutrition and Athletic Performance*
Elson M. Haas, MD and Buck Levin, PhD, RD: *Staying Healthy with Nutrition*
Dr. Edward Howell: *Enzyme Nutrition*
Dr. T.C. Fry and David Klein: *Your Natural Diet*
Paul Nison: *The Raw Life*
Pamela Peeke, MD, MPH: *Fight Fat After Forty*
David Wolfe: *The Sunfood Diet Success System*

HORMONE HEAVEN: Bioidentical Hormones
Russell Roby, JD, MD: *Maybe It IS All in Your Head...and You Are NOT Crazy!*

FENG SHUI
Karen Rauch Carter: *Move Your Stuff, Change Your Life*
Terah Kathryn Collins: *The Western Guide to Feng Shui* and *The Western Guide to Feng Shui: Room by Room*
Karen Kingston: *Clear Your Clutter with Feng Shui*

RESOURCES

Chakra Healing and Therapy
Lisa Powell-Watts, MEd
Licensed Professional Counselor; Graduate, Dr. Brenda Davies
International School of Healing
Spiritual Development
Integration of Psychotherapy and Chakra Healing
Austin, TX
979-830-0960
lisa.pwatts@gmail.com

EFT Therapy
Kay Christopher, LPT, EFT Cert-II
Licensed Pastoral Therapist & Certified EFT Practitioner
(Certified by EFT Founder Gary Craig)
2720 Bee Caves Rd.
Austin, TX 78746
512-358-0770
www.eft-austin.com

EMDR Therapy
Susan Manning
1211 Baylor
Austin, TX 78703
512-320-8001

Energy Healing
Whole Heart & Soul
Tamie Stewart
Shamanic Healing Services
Soul retrieval, ceremony, wellness classes: Shamanic Journey, Shamanic Ritual, How to Be Present in Your Body, Structural Integrity, Structural Bodywork
www.tamiestewart.com
512-294-4605
tamiestewart@ymail.com

Equine Therapy
Sandra DuBose
Program Facilitator
Equine Assisted Learning & Wellness
horseandhealing@yahoo.com
Kerville, TX

Feng Shui
Jillian Lambert
512-965-4252
http://realhealthreallife.net
healthygirl2@gmail.com

Herbalist
Trina Shore Sims
Greenstar Herbs
www.greenstarherbs.com
(512) 301-5069

Intuitive Counselor
Carol Joyce
www.caroljoyce@live.com
505-884-4533

Personal Growth
Millennium 3 Education
Dallas, TX
www.millennium3education.com

Spiritual Coaching
Kellie Jetter CSC, CPLC, CGDP
Soul Coach
Individual Coaching, Workshops & Retreats
www.kelliejetter.com
https://facebook.com/kelliejettersoulcoach

Numerologist
Diane Parma, Numerologist
http://lifebynumbers.com/
512-797-3167
dparma@lifebynumbers.com

Wellness/Chiropractor

Gateway to Wellness

2051 Cypress Creek Rd;

Suite K

Cedar Park, TX 78613

512-250-2224

http://www.g2wchiropractic.com

Wellness/Healing

Georgy Pancharian

Reiki Master

Aromatherapist

www.reikicenteraustin.com

Wellness/Hormones

The Roby Institute

5000 Bee Caves Road

Suite 100

Austin, TX 78746

800-842-6349

http://robyinstitute.com

http://drroby.com

Wellness/Yoga

Susan Anderson

Yoga Wellness Coach

www.happyspineyoga.com

Retreats
Real Health, Real Life Retreat
Fitness, Nutrition, Wellness
Leander, TX
Jillian Lambert, M.S.
http://realhealthreallife.net
healthygirl2@gmail.com
512-965-4252

Silver Spur Ranch
Bandera, TX
www.silverspur-ranch.com
830-796-3037

Travaasa *(Austin and in Hana Hawaii)*
13500 Farm to Market Road 2769
Austin, TX 78726
512-258-7243
855-868-7282
www.travaasa.com

AUTHOR BIO

Jillian Lambert, Nutritionist/Trainer/Consultant/Wellness Expert/
Author

B.S. in Psychology, M.S. in Holistic Nutrition

Jillian Lambert, M.S., is a holistic nutritionist, fitness/wellness
consultant and author. She has worked with spas as an AFAA certified
fitness instructor, personal trainer, holistic nutritionist, feng shui,
emotional health and wellness consultant. Jillian has implemented
fitness, nutrition, weight loss, detox/cleansing and emotional health
programs for various clients over the past 23 years. She is certified in
various areas of fitness ranging from kickboxing and cycling to aqua
and rebounding.

Jillian's background also includes experience in bio-identical
hormones, internal cleansing/detox and years of personal growth
trainings. Being a certified feng shui consultant, Jillian also helps
people detox their homes and offices to create positive energy and
new opportunities in their lives.

In addition to her M.S. in holistic nutrition, Jillian also holds a certification in Living/Raw Foods and a bachelor's in Psychology.

Jillian Lambert
cell: 512-965-4252
http://realhealthreallife.net

healthygirl2@gmail.com

Appendix: Handouts

REAL HEALTH TIPS HANDOUT

*One banana has more electrolytes than a gallon of Gatorade.

*Fatigue can be from not drinking enough water. Take the number of pounds you weigh and divide it in half. That's how many ounces of water you should be drinking each day.

*One serving of alcohol can slow your metabolism for twenty-four hours.

*Newly gained flexibility from stretching is maintained for 1 week and is lost if not maintained.

*Newly gained strength from strength training is maintained for two weeks. The strength gains you made are lost completely after six weeks if not maintained.

*Sleep deprivation can slow down your metabolism. Get some ZZZZZZZs.

*Studies have shown that stretching your muscles in between sets/exercises improves muscle strength.

*Every time you say or think a positive thought, the neurons in your brain reinforce it, making your brain believe it more and more. The same goes for negative thoughts, so think and speak positive!

*Sunshine exposure can help *prevent* breast, colon, ovarian, and prostate cancers.

*If your diet is *low-fat* and contains a lot of fresh fruits, vegetables, and grains, sunlight is *beneficial* to the body.

*Eating a 100 percent raw food diet can improve one's eyesight, arthritis, and many other ailments.

*Organic foods have more vitamins and minerals than conventionally grown foods.

*The essential fatty acids in avocados help you burn unwanted fat!

*Holding your stretches for ten seconds or longer allows oxygen into your muscles, which helps to rebuild them better and stronger.

*Raising your arms overhead while doing aerobics increases your heart rate 30 percent.

*Using free weights helps to increase the strength of your non-dominant side, making both sides more equal in strength.

*Too much protein can create an acidic environment in your body, which can leach calcium from your bones.

*Eating fruit until noon every day helps to cleanse your body internally, frees up energy and possibly help you lose weight. (Detox symptoms may occur within the first one to three days, so give this way of eating at least seven to ten days for best results.)

*Mental strength creates physical strength, so tell yourself you're strong, lean, and healthy.

*Watermelon is the best detoxifier of the fruit family, but eat it on an empty stomach.

*Fruits have the highest amount of vitamins and is second highest in minerals.

*Vegetables have the highest amount of minerals and are second highest in vitamins.

*The seeds on strawberries have ellagic acid inside them, which helps prevent cancer. Break open the seeds with your teeth when chewing and get more out of your strawberries!

*Eating only fresh pears on an empty stomach in the mornings helps your body to eliminate.

*Fresh spinach also stimulates the bowels and helps with elimination.

REAL ENERGY handout

Energy Zappers

* Poor nutrition
* Physical stress
* Emotional stress
* Sleep problems
* Excess travel
* Excess work
* Weather and rain
* Overeating
* Unhealthy foods
* Some times of day
* EMFs *(electromagnetic fields)*
* Dehydration
* Negative people
* Dieting
* Illness
* Depression
* Hormone imbalance
* Some types of food

* Alcohol
* Constipation

ENERGIZERS

1. **Exercise.** Exercise helps improve blood flow to the muscles and brain. Oxygen helps to energize the body as a whole.

2. **Drink Lots of Water.** If your body is dehydrated, you may suffer from fatigue. Take the number of pounds you weigh and divide in half. That's how many ounces of water you should drink daily.

3. **Fruit.** Fruits, especially sweet fruits, provide more energy-fueling sugar: natural sugar. Eat only fruit in the morning, on an empty stomach. Fruit takes very little energy to digest. This leaves more energy left over for you to do other things like exercise or go to work.

4. **Eat proteins with vegetables, not with starchy foods.** Different enzymes digest proteins and starches. Difficult digestion takes more energy from your body, leaving you tired.

5. **Nature.** Nature IS energy. It energizes our bodies, minds and spirits. Experience the trees, rocks, and streams and the breeze across your face, and see how you feel. Nature is one of the true, free energizers we take for granted. Get at least 15 minutes daily.

6. **Balanced Hormones.** Once your hormones are balanced, everything falls into place. Get a simple blood test done and see what hormone balancing can do for you! (Bioidentical hormones are recommended.)

7. **Eat light.** Light snacks and meals are easier to digest. Easier digestion means more energy for you! Overeating can zap your energy and be hard on your digestive system.

8. **Sunshine.** The sun is healing in moderate amounts. It is the best source of vitamin D and increases our sense of wellbeing. Let the sun shine in!

9. **Sleep.** The amount of sleep you get affects your metabolism and energy level. Get to bed earlier. The hours slept before midnight are more restful than the hours following. Go to bed at 9:00 p.m. and see how you feel!

10. **Breathe.** Oxygen. Get oxygen to your lungs, blood, and muscles. Take long, deep breaths whenever you can.

11. **Colonics.** Cleansing the colon can be a great energizer for the body. It can even help people lose weight!

12. **S-t-r-e-t-c-h.** Yoga includes deep breathing and stretching. Holding each stretch for ten seconds or longer allows oxygen to get into the muscles and energize you.

13. **Positive, upbeat people.** Some people are just good energy. You know they are when you feel good and uplifted after being around them.

14. **Feelings of Success.** Anytime we succeed at something, we tend to become energized—even though we may have previously been tired. Success inspires us to keep going.

15. **Other energizers.** Aromatherapy, upbeat music, massage, bright colors.

CALCIUM FOODS handout

Foods are listed from most to least calcium content within each category.

Note: Dairy (Swiss, jack, cheddar, and other cheeses; yogurt, goat's milk, cow's milk) are not recommended because they are considered high acid foods. When the body becomes too acidic health issues may arise and possibly contribute to osteoporosis.
Recommended foods are dark leafy green vegetables, which are high alkaline foods as well as a good calcium source.

Veggies
Broccoli
Collard greens
Turnip greens
Parsley

Nuts/Seeds
Almonds
Brazil nuts
Soybeans

Sunflower seeds
Sesame seeds

Fish
Sardines (with bones)
Salmon (with bones)

Miscellaneous
Molasses
Corn tortilla
Tofu
Dried figs
Dried apricots
Kelp
Soy milk

IRON FOODS handout

Tip: This handout was created for those who are deficient in iron and are looking to include more iron in their diet.

Heme iron in foods is more readily absorbed than iron from non-heme foods. If you eat non-heme iron foods with vitamin C, it helps your body absorb iron. *Heme* means "blood," so iron from animal foods is *heme iron*, while *non-heme* iron comes from plant-based foods.

Beans/legumes (non-heme)

Tofu

Pinto beans

Black beans

Lentils

Peanut butter

Soybeans

Peas

Fruits (with both iron and Vitamin C)

Raisins

Dried apricots

Peaches

Prunes

Figs

Pears

Vegetables (with both iron and Vitamin C)

Tomato juice   Turnips
Collard greens   Winter squash

Grains (non-heme)
Whole wheat   Brown rice
Bread

Meat (heme)
Beef
Liver
Chicken
Turkey
Fish
Pork

JUICING TIPS handout

*Fresh juice has live enzymes, vitamins, and minerals and puts life into your body.

*Store-bought juice is dead juice and puts nothing but calories in your body.

*Drinking fresh juice allows your body to absorb 90 percent of the nutrients.

*Eating fresh fruits and vegetables allows only 10 percent of the nutrients to be absorbed.

*Drinking fresh juice immediately after juicing gives you the most medicinal benefits. This allows your body to absorb the nutrients before the oxidation process sets in.

*Leafy greens are best rolled into a ball and pushed through a juicer with a carrot.

*Pears and peaches (pit removed) are best juiced with alternating apple pieces.

**For best digestive results, fruits and vegetables should really not be juiced together. Apples are the only fruit that can be juiced with vegetables.*

**Lettuce and celery are the only vegetables that can be juiced with fruits.*

*When preparing grapefruit, oranges, tangerines, lemons or limes, cut the colored layer away but leave the white pithy part of the peel. This should be juiced because it is full of bio-flavonoids (plant chemicals).

*Bio-flavonoids help the body absorb vitamin C.

*Cabbage juice helps peptic ulcers but needs to be drunk within one minute of juicing, or all medicinal properties are lost.

*90 percent of the nutrients in a cantaloupe are in the rind. Cantaloupe and watermelon are the most nutritious fruits and are the best detoxifiers of the fruits—rind and all. (Remember to use organic when juicing the rinds.)

*Cucumber is one of the best vegetable detoxifiers and is great for the skin.

*Spinach is one of the most nutritious vegetables when juiced. Spinach juice also helps the body with elimination.

*Ginger in your juice helps with motion sickness and kills parasites. It also helps alleviate nausea and stomach problems associated with pregnancy.

*The calcium in parsley is not absorbed into the body unless it is juiced.

*Pineapple juice has bromelain, which is good for the joints.

*When drinking strawberry juice, make sure to bite into the little seeds. They contain ellagic acid, which help prevent cancer.

*Drink fresh lemon juice with water first thing in the morning to cleanse your liver.

*Drinking fresh pear juice on an empty stomach helps elimination.

*When juicing bitter greens like kale, spinach, or broccoli, fill only one-quarter of your glass with bitter green juice. Fill remainder of glass with milder greens like lettuce, celery, cucumber, and/or apple. This provides many nutrients and is more palatable.

*Sweet fruits such as grapes can be too much sugar for a diabetic person. Be sure to consult with your doctor before adding juicing to your eating program.

*Juicing grapefruit, oranges, and lemons (diluted with water) is a great way to cleanse the body internally.

*Lettuce juice helps to heal/repair the lungs.

*One glass of carrot juice gives you 50 percent of the U.S. Recommended Daily Allowance of Vitamin A.

*When not juicing, chew your food long and well. You'll receive more nutrients.

Note: *To make digestion easier and get the most nutrients from food, chew each bite 50 times.*

CLEANSE/DETOX
MENU handout

3 STAGES OF THE BODY'S DIGESTION SYSTEM WITHIN 24 HOURS
1. Appropriation: Food input/digestion (12:00 noon–8:00 p.m.)
2. Assimilation: Nutrient absorption (8:00 p.m.–4:00 a.m.)
3. Elimination: Waste product elimination (4:00 a.m.–12 Noon)

DETOXIFICATION
Estimated 1-4 days if healthy diet and lifestyle
Estimated 5-10 days if unhealthy diet and lifestyle

POSSIBLE DETOX SYMPTOMS
*Fatigue
*Headache
*Nausea
*Irritability

*Diarrhea

*Light-headedness

Sample menu for 1–2 weeks prior to cleanse:

BREAKFAST

Lemon water upon rising

Fresh, whole, raw fruit and/or fresh juice (preferably organic
fruit)

Any fresh fruit (except dried fruit), throughout morning

LUNCH

Organic Vegetarian Sandwich

> 2 slices Ezekiel Organic Sprouted Grain Bread
>
> 1/2 ripe avocado (may substitute flaxseed oil or coconut oil)
>
> Organic tomato slices
>
> Organic baby carrots cut in half (length-wise)
>
> Organic cucumber slices (skin cut off unless organic)
>
> Organic yellow bell pepper slices (1/4–1/3 section of bell
> pepper)
>
> 2–3 organic romaine lettuce leaves
>
> (Or other variety of fresh, raw vegetables)

Lightly toast Ezekiel bread. Spread avocado or oil onto toast and
top with vegetables.

-OR-

PROTEIN LUNCH

Organic Turkey Wraps (may substitute with lean ground
beef, chicken or tuna)

> 4–6 fresh, organic romaine lettuce leaves
>
> 3–5 oz. free-range, hormone-free lean cooked turkey

organic vegetable mix: 2–3 preferably raw green vegetables
(or lightly steamed)

Wash lettuce leaves. Use each leaf like a taco shell, filling
with turkey and raw veggies.

DINNER

Salmon Salad (may substitute any lean meat such as lean ground
beef, turkey, or chicken)

3-5 oz. of Atlantic salmon

Mrs. Dash seasoning (or your choice of healthy seasoning)

organic spring salad mix

Raw or lightly steamed GREEN veggies (broccoli, green beans,
etc.)

Sprinkle Mrs. Dash or healthy seasoning on salmon. Bake or broil
until cooked thoroughly. Slice or chop salmon and arrange over spring
salad mix.

2-DAY DETOX/CLEANSE HANDOUT

6 large grapefruit

8 large oranges (or tangerines)

4 lemons

1 gallon of purified water.

1 juicer/juice extractor (Juiceman Juicer, Champion, etc.)

With a knife, cut away the surface of the outside peels of the grapefruit, oranges, and lemons.

Be sure to leave the white pithy part of the peel on the fruit. The white pithy part of the peel has bio-flavonoids (plant chemicals) which help with absorption of the vitamin C in the citrus fruit. After cutting away the outside peels, cut fruit in quarters and put through juicer. Make sure you have a large enough container under the juicer to hold the juice. After juicing all the quartered pieces of citrus fruit, mix with ½ gallon of purified water. (If you want the juice to last longer, mix with 1 whole gallon of purified water.)

Keep refrigerated. Drink 8 oz. every hour (instead of food) from morning until evening. Do this for 2 days. Select a 2 day period when you have a light schedule to do a cleanse. Light exercise is okay, just don't overdo it. Please listen to your body. Consult a health care professional before doing any type of cleanse. Be prepared for possible detox symptoms.

LESS WEIGHT handout

Remember two things:1. Water

Drink it. It cleanses the body. It flushes out what your body does not need.

2. **Fiber**

Eat it. Fiber is like taking a scrub brush to the inside of your body. It cleanses your body.

Fat Cells

     Lipogenic (fat-storing enzymes)
     Lipolytic (fat-burning enzymes)
Fat Cells ON: (issues that cause the body to store fat)

1. Dieting/Fasting
2. Lack of sleep
3. Overeating
4. Alcohol
5. Emotional issues

Fat Cells OFF: (things that will help you burn fat off of your body)

1. Exercise
2. Eating small meals
3. Eating often (small meals and snacks)
4. Eating enough
5. Sleep (seven to nine hours)

FRUIT UNTIL NOON handout

WHY FRUIT UNTIL NOON?
*Cleanses internally

*Frees up energy

*Potential weight loss

*Better elimination

*Easy

INTERESTING FACTS ABOUT BANANAS
*Bananas are a healthy carb and contain healthy sugars. (Energy requires sugar.)

*Bananas contain healthy sugars that are lost after an exercise workout, so eat a banana after you exercise.

*One banana has more electrolytes than a gallon of sports drink.

*90 minutes of exercise causes loss of electrolytes, and bananas can help restore electrolyte levels.

BANANA BENEFITS (WHEN EATEN ON AN EMPTY STOMACH)

*Instant energy

*Sustained energy

*High in iron

*Helps blood pressure

*High in potassium

*Boosts brain power

*Helps constipation

*Helps to relax

*#1 fruit with world athletes

*High in fiber

*Helps with anemia

*Reduces risk of stroke

*Low in salt

*Increases alertness

*Helps depression

*Improves mood

Note: *Only eat bananas on an empty stomach.*

PARTY EATING handout

We all love a party…whether it's the fun, the relaxation, or the food. Parties can be healthy, too, if you keep the following tips in mind:

* Bring a veggie tray or something else healthy to the party.
This way you will always have something healthy to eat.

*Eat something healthy before leaving for the party.
You'll eat less food at the party.

*Drink water BEFORE eating at the party.
Don't mistake hunger for thirst.

*Stay away from white, starchy foods…especially late in the day or evening.

*Ask coworkers to put holiday "goodies" on the other side of the office.
Out of sight, out of mind. Tell them you don't want to gain the "Holiday 7."

* **Stay out of the kitchen at parties. Take conversations to another room.**

People tend to hang out in the kitchen at parties and eat more when surrounded by food.

***Cut back on alcohol.**

One serving of alcohol slows your metabolism down for twenty-four hours.

Beverage	Calories	Amount
Eggnog	343	8 oz./1 cup
Apple cider	116	8 oz./1 cup
Wine (red)	144	8 oz./1 cup
Wine (white)	150	8 oz/1 cup

***Eat enough fruit in the morning (on an empty stomach).**

This helps you stave off sweet cravings later in the day or evening.

***Eat protein, not carbs, in the evening.**

Get enough carbs—healthy carbs (like fruit)—early in the day so you don't overdo it at the party.

Protein	Calories	Amount
Beef brisket (lean)	298	2 medium slices, 123 g
Baked ham	254	2 medium slices, 156 g
Roasted turkey	128	2 medium slices, 75g
Shrimp cocktail	8 (per large shrimp w/o sauce)	

***Love yourself *more* than you love the food.**

RESTAURANT EATING handout

You can go hog wild at a restaurant and eat whatever you want, or you can keep a few tips in mind that will help you feel better, healthier, and help you avoid putting on extra weight.

1. **Order your water with lemon slices.** Squeeze lemon into water. Lemon water helps hold off hunger temporarily. You'll be less likely to grab for the bread or chips. They are high in fat, high in calories, and low in nutrients.
2. **Drink 8–12 oz. of water 10 minutes before your meal.** You will hydrate yourself and not mistake thirst for a hunger pang. Drinking water prior to your meal will also make you eat less food.
3. **Order a salad with your meal**. You'll consume fewer calories and more fiber. The enzymes in the raw vegetables also help digest the other cooked (or less healthy) food in your meal.
4. **Order your salad dressing on the side.** Many restaurants *drench* their salads with dressing and *you* pay the price. Most

restaurants want the food to taste good, not to be low in calories.

5. **Dip your fork into salad dressing prior to each bite. Don't pour it over your salad.** You will use less dressing, getting fewer calories and less fat.

6. **Move the bread basket and salsa chips *away* from you or *off* the table.** Bread will fill you up, but it is high in calories and low in nutrients. Tortilla chips are high in fat and calories, but low in nutrients. Try salsa and celery.

7. **Order your food baked, broiled, or grilled.** Trans fats from fried foods are not recognized by the body and are stored as fat.

8. **Order your protein with steamed vegetables or a salad.** Eating starchy carbs at night will only add to your weight. Starchy carbs are usually white foods like pasta, bread, rice, potatoes, or desserts

9. **Order sauces on the side. Dip fork into the sauce and spread it *lightly* over your entrée.** This way your entrée is not drenched in high calories and fat.

10. ***Do not* view the dessert tray.** Visual stimulation only increases desire for high fat/high carb desserts. Why do you think the waiter brings the dessert tray to your table? It is much easier to say no to something you *don't* see.

11. **If you must have a dessert, split it with someone or eat fewer bites.** Eating enough fruit early in the day on an empty stomach will help decrease later cravings for sweets.

12. **Do *not* overeat!** Listen to your body. *Stop* when full. Overeating causes excess weight and poor digestion. Any calories over the 500 mark at one sitting are more likely to be stored as fat.

ALLERGY DIET handout

Food Restrictions

Stay away from these food groups during air-borne allergy season to eliminate allergy symptoms such as sinus congestion, sinus pressure, runny nose, sinus headache, itchy ears and throat, itchy feet and hands, and so on. If you'd like to test this diet, restrict these particular foods for five days. After five days, eat one of your favorite foods to discover which food(s) you are sensitive to.

> *Citrus fruits: grapefruit, oranges, tangerines, clementines, tangelos, lemons, limes. Pineapple is also an acid fruit and therefore restricted.
>
> *Dairy foods: pasteurized cow's milk, cheese, yogurt, cottage cheese
>
> *Tomatoes: tomatoes, tomato sauce, salsa, etc.
>
> *Grains: wheat, rice, pasta
>
> *Chocolate
>
> *Dark colas (light colored diet sodas are permitted)
>
> *Sugar
>
> *Eggs

ALLERGY DIET SAMPLE

This is a sample list of foods and food combinations to eat on a day during allergy season.

*Apples, bananas, peaches, pears, papaya, melons, etc.
*Avocado and romaine lettuce (avocado lettuce wraps)
*Tuna and romaine lettuce (tuna lettuce wraps)
*Broccoli and turkey

Note: *The allergy diet is from Dr. Roby's book*

YOU CAN EAT:

Non-citrus fruits
Vegetables (except tomatoes)
Turkey
Chicken
Beef
Fish
Water (woo-hoo!)

REAL RECIPES handout (5 ingredients or less)

Preparing food can be time-consuming and unhealthy, or it can be quick, easy and healthy. Here are some recipes that I have created and used over the years. Some recipes are vegetarian, some are not. They combine foods properly to help with digestion and free up energy! Each recipe has five ingredients or less: quick, easy, and healthy!

REAL JUICES (You'll need a juicer)

CARROT-APPLE JUICE
> 1 apple (no core)
> 2 carrots

Juice ingredients and drink immediately after juicing. The longer fresh juice sits out, the quicker it oxidizes and loses its medicinal value. Nutrients are being lost every minute that the juice sits out. Refrigeration helps somewhat.

GRAPE-LEMON-APPLE JUICE

    1 bunch of grapes (red or green)

    1/4 lemon (with peel)

    1 apple (no core)

Juice all ingredients. Drink with a little umbrella in glass to make more tropical!

REAL PROTEIN SHAKE (Tofu)

    1/2 to 1 whole 12.3-oz. carton Mori-Nu Lite (or regular) Tofu, FIRM

    4–6 large (or 6–9 small) Medjool dates (soaked overnight for better digestion)

    1 banana

    3–4 ice cubes

    1/4 cup purified water

    Make sure there are no pits in the dates. Blend all ingredients together, including water from the soaking dates. If it is not sweet enough, add 1–2 more dates. Enjoy!

REAL ALMOND SHAKE

    3/4 cup raw almonds

    4–5 large (or 6–9 small) Medjool dates

    1 banana (optional)

    3–4 ice cubes

    1/4 cup purified water

    Soak almonds overnight in clean water. It is much healthier for you if the almonds are soaked first, because that releases the enzyme inhibitors and makes for easier digestion.

    Drain water and rinse almonds before blending, and

make sure there are no pits in the dates. Blend all ingredients together. For chunky consistency, blend a short amount of time. For smooth consistency, blend longer. If not sweet enough, add 1–2 more dates. Enjoy!

BANAN-ADE (great for after a workout)

    1–2 bananas

    12–16 oz. purified water

Blend 1 or 2 bananas and water in a blender. This drink will replace any electrolytes that may have been lost through exercise or stress. (One banana has more electrolytes than a gallon of sports drink.)

REAL QUICK SNACKS / MINI-MEALS:

Real Rainbow Sandwich (*more than 5 ingredients depending how many vegetables*)

    Ezekiel Bread (sprouted grain bread)

    Tomato

    Cucumber

    Baby carrots

    Romaine lettuce

    Alfalfa sprouts (or other kind of sprouts)

    Yellow bell pepper (or red or orange, though yellow has the most vitamin C)

    Flax seed oil (can substitute sliced avocado or coconut oil)

Lightly toast the bread. Pour a small amount of flax seed oil on it. Place all cut-up veggies on bread. Eat a Real Rainbow of veggies!

Avocado Tacos

    1 large avocado

    1/2 tomato (optional)

1/4 cucumber (optional)

Romaine heart lettuce head (Earth Bound Farm Organic Romaine Hearts is what I use)

1 container of Ana's Salsa (mild, medium, or hot)

Cut open avocado. Remove pit/stone. Scoop out avocado flesh and place in bowl. Mix in salsa. If you want more veggies, add tomato and cucumber.

Once mixed together, scoop out and place inside romaine leaf. Lettuce leaf will be like a taco shell, but healthier. Eat like a taco!

ROMAINE WRAPS

3–5 oz. of turkey, tuna, chicken (roasted, baked, or broiled—*not* fried) or steak

5–10 romaine lettuce leaves

Small amount of diced tomatoes or cucumbers (optional)

Place your choice of meat or fish (and tomatoes if desired) inside a romaine lettuce leaf, using it like a taco shell. The lettuce gives you something healthy and crunchy, with enzymes to help digest the filling!

Tuna Salad Filling Variation:

1 can of tuna (water packed)

1 tbsp of Nayonaise (tofu mayonnaise, the healthier option) or 1 tbsp of mayonnaise

1–2 stalks of celery and/or cucumbers (diced)

Drain water from tuna. Mix the tuna, Nayonaise, or mayonnaise, and celery together and spoon into lettuce leaves.

EGG WRAPS

3–5 oz. of scrambled eggs

5–10 romaine lettuce leaves

1 handful of mozzarella cheese or raw cheese for added enzymes (optional)

2–3 tbsp. salsa (optional)

Place scrambled eggs inside a romaine lettuce leaf, using it like a taco shell. Sprinkle a small amount of cheese and salsa on the eggs, or just salsa (this, of course, is the healthier choice). This adds a bit of flavor to your egg wrap. The enzymes in the lettuce and salsa help digest the eggs.

TOFU BROCCOLI

Broccoli (*lightly* steamed)

Tofu (*lightly* steamed)

1/4 or 1/2 lemon (optional)

Mix broccoli with tofu. The crunchier the broccoli remains, the more enzymes for your body. To add some flavor, squeeze lemon over the dish.

Note: *Don't forget to take an enzyme capsule BEFORE your meal. Even though the food is only lightly steamed, it IS considered cooked…healthy, but cooked!*

PEANUT-APPLE SNACK

1–2 tbsp. of real peanut butter (the ingredients are just peanuts—*no* hydrogenated oils)

1 sliced apple

Spread the peanut butter on the apple slices (or dip the apples into the peanut butter). This is a good food combination and includes protein and a Real carb. A healthy treat!

Almond Butter Variation: Use almond butter instead of peanut butter.

ORANGE ALMONDS

> 1 orange
> 1 handful of raw almonds

Eat the orange, then the almonds in that order (for MUCH better digestion). This is another snack that provides a protein and a Real carb.

DATED ALMOND TREAT

> 5–10 almonds
> 5-10 Medjool dates (pitted)

Remove pit from dates and insert almonds. This is a deliciously sweet, yet crunchy treat!

BROCCOLI SALMON (my all-time favorite meal)

> 1 salmon fillet
> ½ bunch of broccoli
> ½ lemon

Broil salmon in oven or broiler. Cook 10-20 min. depending on size of fillet. Steam broccoli on high for 5-6 minutes, still leaving it crunchy. Cut ½ lemon and squeeze over cooked salmon fillet and broccoli.

Eat and enjoy! Very healthy

That's it! Eat up! Happy digestion!

STRENGTH TRAINING handout

BENEFITS:
*stronger bones

*stronger muscles

*stronger connective tissue

*improves physical ability

*prevents injuries

*increases metabolism

GUIDELINES:
*Start with a warm-up to increase body temperature (walking, marching, etc.)

*8–12 repetitions with weights that are somewhat challenging

*3 sets if time allows. If not, do 1 set. (1 set gives 92 percent of the benefits of doing 3)

*Start with large muscle groups, then move to small muscle groups

*Move weight with a 95 percent range of motion

*Exhale on the exertion part of the movement (Blow out on the hard part of exercise.)

*Slower is better. Slower is more challenging. Slower is more effective. Slower is safer.

*Give muscles a rest between sessions (forty-eight hours rest for each muscle group worked)

*End your workout with stretches, or stretch the muscles worked between each set. Hold each stretch for at least ten seconds. This allows oxygen to get in and rebuilds the muscles better and stronger.

RECOMMENDED STRENGTH TRAINING EXERCISES:

Exercise	Muscle Group
Leg press	Quads, Glutes (front thighs, butt)
Leg curl	Hamstrings (back thighs)
Chest press	Pectorals, deltoids, triceps
Lat pull-down	Lats (back)
Row	Trapezius (upper back)
Overhead press	Deltoids (shoulders)
Overhead extension	Triceps (upper back arms)
Arm curl	Biceps (front mid arms)
Crunches	Abdominals (upper abs)
Back extension	Erector Spinae (back)

STABILITY BALL handout

BENEFITS:

    *Improves balance

    *Strengthens abdominal muscles

    *Strengthens back muscles

    *Total body workout

    *Improves body awareness

    *Makes exercise more fun!

GUIDELINES:

    *Make sure you maintain proper air pressure in the ball. When it is firm, the exercises are more difficult. When the ball is soft, the exercises are easier.

    *Size does make a difference. Knees and hips should form a 90-degree angle when you are seated on the ball. Appropriate ball sizes according to height are listed below.

Height	Ball Size
*5'0" tall and under	45 cm ball
*5'0"–5'7"	55 cm ball
*5'8"–6'2"	65 cm ball
*6'2" and taller	75 cm ball

SERENITY
S-T-R-E-T-C-H handout

Stretching is beneficial for the body, mind and spirit. Stretching your muscles is vital to keep them supple. Regular stretching helps keep your body strong and functional.

BENEFITS:
*Improves muscle strength

*Increases range of motion

*Improves posture

*Rejuvenates/revitalizes body, mind, spirit

*Improves muscle function

*Oxygenates muscles

*Keeps muscles supple

*Decreases likelihood of injury

*Decreases stress

GUIDELINES:

*Stretch only up to where it feels good, never to where it hurts

*Hold all stretches at least ten seconds to reap the benefits

*After holding stretch for ten seconds or longer, the muscle relaxes and allows oxygen into the muscles to help rebuild it better and stronger

*Initially, the muscle tightens up while being stretched. A defense mechanism called the *stretch reflex* tightens the muscle to protect itself from injury (being overstretched). Holding a stretch for at least ten seconds gives a muscle time to realize it is not going to be overstretched.

*Cancer cells cannot survive in an environment with oxygen, so hold your stretches and allow oxygen to get into all muscles from all angles.

*Stretching is recommended every day. If you are not able to stretch daily, 3–4 times per week will keep your body flexible and you'll reap the many benefits stretching affords.

*Stretching a minimum of once a week is necessary in order to keep the gains you have made in flexibility. Otherwise, all gains are lost.

*Everybody's flexibility is different. Your right side may be more flexible than your left or vice versa. That's normal, but it is very important to aim for balance in your flexibility (with your right side as flexible as your left and your front as flexible as your back).

METABOLISM MISTAKES handout

Exercising too much. Excess exercise slows down the metabolism; it makes the body cling to remaining fat as a survival mechanism. The body wants to make sure that there is enough fat to keep it warm and the organs protected.

Genetics. Genetics may determine whether you have a fast or slow metabolism, but you can increase it with a few tweaks in movement, nutrition, and lifestyle.

Inactivity. A sedentary lifestyle will give you the metabolism of a snail unless you are blessed genetically.

Sleep deprivation. Lack of sleep will make your fat burning process much slower and less efficient. Sleep is soooooo important! Get seven to nine hours, or until you wake up naturally without an alarm clock.

Skipping meals. Skipping meals can lead your body into starvation mode. Since the body does not know when its next meal/calories are coming, it needs to conserve energy, thereby rationing the calories burned. This slows the body's metabolism.

P.M. Exercise. Exercising in the evening gives your metabolism a boost, but only for a short while. Your metabolism is already slowing down for the day. If that's the best time to exercise for you, by all means, go for it. It will still help—just not as much as exercising in the morning.

P.M. Eating. Eating right before bed makes people more likely to have nightmares. Not only does the body not have enough time to digest the calories before falling asleep, but evening metabolism is also slower. It's your body's way of winding down for the night. Those calories can be stored as fat if not properly digested.

Dieting. Extreme changes in the way you eat can mess with your metabolism. The "roller-coaster" way of eating can shift your metabolism in and out of survival mode, causing your metabolism to slow down.

Not eating enough calories. Depriving yourself of necessary calories your body needs lowers your metabolism. Lack of calories tells the body that there may not be enough food in the future, so it tends to burn them more slowly.

Alcohol. One serving of alcohol (one beer, glass of wine, or a mixed drink) slows the metabolism down for a minimum of twenty-four hours after you drink it. Also, the body processes the alcohol calories before food calories.

Age. Metabolism tends to slow down as we age, but we can get around that by keeping active and following other metabolism booster tips.

Overeating. Eating too much food at a time can cause the body to store excess calories as fat.

Unbalanced hormones. Once your hormones are balanced, there's a better chance of everything else in the body being balanced. A simple blood test can tell you where you stand regarding hormone levels.

METABOLISM BOOSTERS handout

Exercise. Any form of exercise speeds up the metabolism, compared to being sedentary. Take the stairs, do some gardening, walk the dog.

Genetics. Some of us are blessed with a fast metabolism. If you have a fast metabolism, enjoy it. Use it to your advantage, but most of all, appreciate it.

Busyness. People who cannot sit still increase their metabolism. All that activity throughout the day adds up. Please don't take this too much to heart, as we are all too busy with life as it is.

Sleep. The proper amount of sleep will make your fat burning process more efficient.

Interval Training. Placing more cardiovascular demands on your body speeds up your metabolism.

Strength Training. Placing more strength demands on your body speeds up your metabolism.

A.M. Exercise. Early morning exercise boosts metabolism and benefits you for the rest of the day.

Mental Activity – Mental activity that stimulates *productive* thought processes helps boost metabolism. The key word is *productive*. Watching TV or playing the same old video games don't count.

Small, frequent meals. Digestion helps to speed the metabolism. It takes a lot of energy for your body to digest food. Digestion takes more energy than it does for running, swimming or bike riding. Eating small, frequent meals keeps the fat burning fires going all day. Just make sure you're eating healthy food or you'll be defeating the whole purpose of speeding up your metabolism.

Time of day you eat. Eating before 8:00 p.m. is important to make the most of digestion and metabolism. There's a saying: "Eat after Eight, Gain Weight." If you *really* want to lose weight, don't eat after 5:00 p.m.

Age. Our metabolism is much faster in our younger years.

Hormones. – Getting your hormones balanced can make a huge difference in your metabolism.

Colonics. Colon cleansing improves the efficiency of your digestive tract and elimination system, giving your metabolism a boost.

Pregnancy. Creating a baby is a lot of work! This whole process increases your metabolism.

Breastfeeding. Generating milk for your baby is also extra work for your body and gives your metabolism a boost.

THINGS TO KEEP IN MIND ABOUT METABOLISM BEFORE EATING:

Protein. Breaking down protein requires more of your body's energy and speeds up metabolism.

Fiber. Digesting fiber gives metabolism a boost.

Calcium. Calcium helps increase metabolism and helps with weight loss.

Spicy foods. Spicy foods increase metabolism temporarily, although not by much. Don't counteract the benefits by eating something fattening. Keep it healthy.

*Note: *Do not take in too much protein or calcium. It can create an acidic environment within the body. If your body becomes too acidic, calcium can be leached from the bones to help neutralize the acid.*

HEALING EFFECTS OF THE SUN handout

Benefits of sun exposure:

    *Sunlit houses can help prevent disease, make us feel happier, and save energy.

    *Sunlight can help prevent and heal many common and often fatal diseases like breast cancer, heart disease, multiple sclerosis and osteoporosis.

    *Before antibiotics, sunlight was used successfully to speed up the healing of wounds

    *Early morning sun (within four hours of sunrise) and early evening sun (within four hours of sunset are the best times for sun exposure.

    *Sun exposure creates the best form of vitamin D.

    *Moderate sunbathing in the spring and early summer is the best time of the year to absorb and store vitamin D.

    *Worldwide, the countries where sunscreens have been recommended and adopted have experienced the greatest rise in malignant melanoma. (U.S., Canada, Australia, and the Scandinavian countries)

*Tanning moderately throughout the year is better than avoiding the sun altogether.

*Sudden bursts of strong solar radiation are can be dangerous, so protection needs to be built up slowly.

*Combining a high-fat, low-nutrient diet and sunlight exposure can have negative effects on your health. For more information see *The Healing Sun* by Richard Hobday.

*Sunlight enters the body through two organs: your skin and your eyes.

*Removing glasses, sunglasses, and/or contacts when outside helps to stimulate the pineal gland.

*Being free of glasses, sunglasses and/or contacts allows sunshine to enter the eyes helping to improve your immune system and vision.

*Early morning sunlight in cool temperatures is particularly beneficial to the body.

*Sunlit hospital rooms provide a better environment for the treatment of clinically depressed people.

*Fluorescent lights emit mercury vapor, 100 times the amount shown on lighting charts. Mercury vapor can cause severe food allergies according to the book *Light: Medicine of the Future*.

*Ergosterol is a sterol within your skin that is activated by sunlight and then turned into vitamin D.

*Large numbers of people may be compromising their health with sunlight deficiency.

*There is a substantial body of historical and contemporary evidence that suggests moderate sunbathing is far more beneficial than we are currently led to believe.

See The Healing Sun: Sunlight and Health in the 21st Century *by Richard Hobday, MSc, PhD and* Light: Medicine of the Future *by Jacob Liberman, OD, PhD*

ANIMAL SYMBOLISM handout

Bear. Trust your inner voice

Bees. Fertility, sexuality, productivity, accomplishing the impossible, enjoying the sweetness of life

Butterfly. Transformation, dancing, joy, lightheartedness, new birth

Blackbird. Promise, protect what you own

Bluebird. Happiness

Canary. Voice, trust your voice

Cardinal. Monogamy, courtship, relationships, feminine side, the number 12, attend to health, self-importance

Cat. Independence, mystery

Cougar. Leadership, strength, staying on track with goals, self-empowerment

Coyote. Trickery, wisdom, trust the plan

Cricket. Good luck, finding light, protection of home, beliefs, trust intuition

Crow. Magical help with problems

Deer. Power of gentleness, innocence, new adventures

Dragonfly. Efforts are coming to fruition, time to shine

Dog. Faithfulness, loyalty, protection of self and surroundings

Dove. Peace, new opportunities

Duck. Emotions to be soothed

Eagle. Vision, spirit, spiritual

Fox. Beware of camouflaged surroundings, do not reveal your plan, shifting situations, magic

Frog. Transformation, emotions, water

Gecko. Take action

Hawk. Guiding vision, observe, opportunities, surrounding guardianship

Horse. Freedom, strength, beauty, grace, power, new journeys ahead

Hummingbird. Joy

Ladybug. Wish fulfilled

Lion. Strength of will

Lizard. Dreams, intuition, pay attention to dreams and psychic feelings

Mouse. Focus on details

Owl. Wisdom, moon, hear what is hidden, spirits

Praying Mantis. Stillness, be patient for success

Rabbit. Overcoming fear, wait for answers

Raccoon. Disguise, masking is happening

Roadrunner. Speed, to think quickly

Scorpion. Transformation, sexual needs, passion

Snake. Rebirth, transformation, healing, protector, shed the old skin

Spider. Weaving fate, trust feeling, not what you see

Squirrel. Gather, prepare, busyness, conserve, work and play

Tiger. Power, assert power

Toad. Emotional cleansing, transformation, inner strength, good luck, money

Turtle. Promise, take your time

Wasp. Protection around you

Wolf. Spirit guide, loyalty, intuition, learning, inner strength, protected, trust in self

To find symbolism of animals not listed, look up the animal you'd like to know about on Google, using its name and the phrase "animal symbolism." *Example: alligator animal symbolism*

HEALING (AND CHAKRA BALANCING) STONES CHART handout

*Agate – good health, helps stomach and ulcers, prosperity, reduces fever, protects, self-clarity, world clarity, helps with sleep and eliminating fear, self-confidence, throat chakra.

*Amber (amber is not actually a stone, but is made of tree resin) – happy, carefree, optimistic, self-confident, powerful, calm, strong, good sense of humor solar plexus chakra.

*Amethyst – spiritual awareness, meditation stone, wisdom, peace, strengthens immunity, peace of mind, cleans blood, protects against drunkenness and negativity, addictions, relieves headaches, improves blood sugar imbalance, brow chakra.

*Aquamarine – mental clarity, improves creativity, reduces stress, courage, strengthens will, protects, re-awakens love, helps with nerve pain, tooth, neck, jaw, throat, eyes ears, stomach, liver, kidney, helps depression and grief, throat chakra.

*Aventurine – self-confidence, patience, relaxation, acceptance, tolerance, improves sleep, heart chakra.

*Bloodstone – magic stone, helps with more knowledge, stops bleeding/hemorrhages with slight touch, helps stomach and intestinal pain, helps with addictions, depression, self-confidence, strengthens blood, root chakra.

*Blue lace agate – calm, centering, throat chakra.

*Calcite – trust, motivation, positivity, solar plexus chakra.

*Carnelian – courage, cheerfulness, calming, voice strengthener, dispels fear, helps with depression, sacral chakra.

*Coral – protector of children, helps with emotional conflict, wisdom, promotes health, helps heal nutritional deficiencies, lungs, digestion, circulation, depression, root chakra. (Broken coral will not help heal.)

***Chrysocolla** – stomach ulcers.

*Chrysoprase – balances emotions, mental and physical, stability, youthfulness, happiness, detoxifies, communication, patience, willpower.

*Citrine – joy, happiness, optimism, openness, prosperity, abundance stone, calming, peace, direction, healing stone, helps w/depression, improves memory, detoxifies body, helps digestion, liver, kidney and heart, solar plexus chakra.

Emerald – physical and emotional healing, faith, wisdom, good fortune, success in love, protect from evil, poison antidote, helps with eyes and spine.

Hematite – healing, grounding, inner peace, helps with venereal disease, bladder.

Garnet – balance, peace, protection, faith, courage, truth, grace, compassion, stimulates sex drive, energizes, health, helps with blood, pituitary gland, arthritis, depression, fidelity, root chakra. Garnet should be worn close to the body.

Fluorite – stand ground, speak up, stimulates learning, integrity, potential fulfillment, throat chakra.

Jade – good fortune, health, wealth, prosperity, regulates heart, longevity, heart chakra.

Labradorite – helps transformation go smoothly, improves sleep, opens solar plexus, brow chakras (and others if needed).

Lapis Lazuli – helps mental clarity, meditation, calmness, promotes psychic skills and spirituality, helps relieve negative emotions/anti-depressant, thyroid, cataracts and sore throats, throat and brow chakra.

Malachite – grounding, business success, vision, reduces confusion, clears obstructions, energizes, calms emotions, deepens compassion and empathy, soothes nervous system, harmonizes life, brings knowledge, patience, helps regenerate cells, calms, improves sleep, and heals past sexual abuse.

*Moonstone – female protection, good fortune, increases passion, helps digestion and vertebrae, balances emotions.

*Onyx – rids self of negative thinking, helps with spirituality, helps change habits, strengthens eyes, nails, hair, nerves, kidneys, heart, improves sleep, reduces stress and apathy, keeps emotions under control, self-control, aligned consciousness.

*Opal – healing of blood, depression, apathy, spleen, pancreas, brain and mental aspects, protection, lucky stone, means faithfulness and confidence.

*Pearl – heals heart chakra, stomach, spleen, intestines and ulcers, improves self-worth, corrects emotional imbalances, symbolizes love, happiness, and success.

*Peridot – healing, makes dreams come true, attracts love, attracts wealth, wards off negativity, improves strength and vitality, soothes hurt feelings, protects, helps sinuses, lungs, and emotions.

*Quartz (clear) – healing stone except for cancer, (do not use if you have or had cancer), stone does not need cleansing, helps cleanse other stones, crown chakra.

*Rhodochrosite – Forgiveness.

*Rose Quartz – love, peace, true love of self and others, heals trauma, releases impurities, heart chakra.

HEALING STONES CHART HANDOUT

*Ruby – power, passion, root chakra.

*Silver – improves speech, belief/faith in self, throat chakra.

*Smoky Quartz – helps release what no longer serves you, neutralizes negativities from self, others, EMFs and environment, replaces with gentle, positive energy, root chakra

*Sodalite – spirituality, truth, objective, detachment, brow chakra.

*Sugilite (luvulite) – strength, stand ground in opinions and beliefs even under pressure, open to working out conflicts, brow chakra.

*Tiger's eye – protection, improves confidence and focus, willpower, healing for kidney, asthma, heart, psoriasis, and blood pressure, solar plexus and sacral chakras.

*Tourmaline – protection from danger, improves creativity, altruism and fertility, rids one of fear and negativity, helps balance hormones, relaxes, and helps with heart disease and arthritis.

*Topaz – balancing, brings joy, spiritual, emotions in balance, helps with tissue, blood, endocrine system and appetite.

*Turquoise – healing, love, friendship, happiness, good fortune, protection, communication, expression, prosperity, emotional balance, helps with all disease, alignment and strength. Warns of danger, attracts healing spirits, throat chakra.

IONIC FOOT BATH CHART handout

Color Chart

Color or Particle	Material or Area of Body
*Yellow-green	Detoxifying from the kidneys, bladder, urinary tract, female/prostate area
*Orange	Detoxifying from joints
*Brown	Detoxifying liver, tobacco, cellular debris
*Black	Detoxifying from liver
*Dark green	Detoxifying from gallbladder and lymphatic system (most likely yeast)

Particles:

*Black flecks	Heavy metals
*Red flecks	Blood cut material

JOURNALING WITH JILLIAN handout

The act of writing can be very therapeutic. Journaling can express our reactions to experiences. It can counteract the negative effects of stress and decrease the symptoms of many health conditions, improve our cognitive functioning, and strengthen our immune system.

Journaling is a very valuable tool to help us express feelings that we may otherwise not express. It is a safe place to put our feelings and to "get them out." Journaling helps us realize what we feel, how we feel, and why we feel it. Writing it out helps us to see things in the third person and to recognize things we may not normally notice. When thoughts are floating around in our head, we are too close to them and there may be a pattern that is difficult to interrupt. Once the thoughts are written down, we can see them for what they are—not what they seem to be.

Overall, journaling heals us.

Journal to:

*Release your anger.

*Release your guilt.

*Release your doubt.

*Release your pain.

See your emotional wounds be healed. Purge the negative and take in the positive.

Let the pain leave your heart. Allow joy and inner peace to replace it.

Write out the bad things in your life. Write in the good. Write your own life script.

See things that you've always wanted come into your life. You can have it all. You can have true love, peace, joy, health, wealth, success, and prosperity...total abundance.

Write it.
You deserve it.

JOURNALING TOPICS TO HELP YOU GET STARTED

I fear_____.

I doubt_____.

I feel guilty about_____.

I feel angry about_____.

I feel pain about_____.

I feel fearful because_____.

I feel doubtful because_____.

I feel guilty because_____.

I feel angry because_____.

I feel pain because_____.

I release my fear of_____.

I release all doubt about_____.

I release my anger about_____.

I release my pain about_____.

I release old negative patterns, such as_____.

I take on new positive patterns, such as_____.

It does not matter what other people say or do. What matters is what I believe about myself.

I believe_____.

I am free to let go of_____.

I am safe to_____.

I am free to_____.

I take responsibility in my life by_____.

My spiritual growth is lifting me to my highest good by_____.

The next step for my highest good is_____.

I give myself permission to let go of_____.

I am_____.

I appreciate my body because_____.
I love my body because_____.
I show my body I love it by_____.
I love_____.
I appreciate_____.
I feel love when_____.
I feel appreciated when_____.
I am grateful to be alive today because_____.

I am discovering new ways to improve my health by_____.
I give my body what it needs on every level. What it needs is_____.
I balance my life equally between work, rest, and play. To make a better
balance,
I will_____.
I am willing to ask for help when I need it. I need help with_____.
I trust my intuition. I listen, trust and act on it.
My intuition says_____.

I feel healthy when_____.
I feel loving when_____.
I feel positive when_____.

I listen to my feelings. I am gentle with myself. My feelings are my friend
and guide. My feelings guide me to_____.

I am forgiving, gentle, and kind.
I forgive everyone in my past for all perceived wrongs. I release them
with love.
I forgive_____.

They did the best they could with the knowledge, understanding, and awareness that they had at the time. I am strong to forgive and let go. I let go of all fear.

I forgive_____.

I forgive myself for_____.

I forgive myself because_____.

I forgive others for_____.

I let go of_____.
The past is over. The power is now. I am powerful. I claim my own power.

I have the power to_____.
I am free from the past. I move into joy.

I feel joy when_____.
I get help from various sources. My support system is strong and loving.

It helps me to _____.

I am living the best way I know how. That way is to_____.

I am making positive changes in all areas of my life like_____.

Money is_____.

I feel this way about money because_____.

I feel my income is_____because_____.

If I had all the money in the world, I would_____.

I prosper wherever I turn. I feel prosperous when_____.

I am open and receptive to all good and abundance in the universe. Thank you, life!

My good and abundance is_____.

I am a magnet for money. Prosperity is drawn to me because_____.
I think big and allow myself to accept even more good from life. More good is_____.
I allow prosperity to enter my life on a higher level than ever before. This higher level looks like_____.
Enormous wealth and abundance are available to me now. I am worthy and deserving of it because _____

We are here to bless and prosper one another. I let others be who they are.
I feel blessed because_____.
I am grateful for the good in my life. The good is_____.

I am creative. I feel creative when_____.
I am creative in everything I do. I created_____.
I am the creator of my life.
I will create_____
I can create anything.

My career is_____.
Success is_____.
My talents are in demand and my unique gifts are appreciated by everyone.
My gifts are_____.
I deserve to have a successful career and I accept it now.
My idea of a successful career is_____.
I am successful at everything I do. I am successful at_____.
My career is_____.
Thank you for bringing me success.

Love is_____.

I love_____.

A relationship is_____.

I am treated like_____because_____.

I am scared to love because_____.

I am scared to *be* loved because_____.

I attract only healthy relationships. I am always treated well.

A healthy relationship is_____.

I would like to be treated like_____.

I love everyone and everything.

I love myself.

I love myself because_____.

I am love.

Thank you for bringing me true love.

I am_____.

SOUL JOURNAL handout

My soul is _____.

My soul wants_____.

My soul says_____.

My soul yearns for_____.

_____makes my soul happy.

_____makes my soul dance.

My body is_____.

My body feels like_____.

My body wants_____.

My body says_____.

My body yearns for_____.

I would like my body to_____.
_____makes my body happy.

The worst thing about my body is_____.

The best thing about my body is_____.

I wish my body_____.

The most incredible thing my body does is_____.

I am grateful for my body's_____.

MIRROR, MIRROR ON THE WALL/POSITIVE AFFIRMATIONS handout

Mirror, Mirror on the Wall...

The mirror reflects much about how we look. It helps us apply makeup, remove something from an eye, see cars to the rear and side of us while driving. It also helps us to view, up close, any and all physical flaws.

The mirror can be an enemy, or it can be a friend.

Looking in the mirror to see your physical self is one thing, but have you ever looked into the mirror to see your emotional self?

It's a whole other world....
Looking at yourself in the mirror does not only reveal physical aspects, assets and imperfections...it can also reveal your emotional soul.

Louise Hay is a woman who experienced a very traumatic life growing up. She was abused physically, emotionally and sexually. Over the years, she found a way to heal her emotional wounds. Not only did she heal her emotions, but she healed her life.

Louise created affirmations. We've all heard of affirmations, you know, the positive statements you say out loud to help you think positive. Sometimes they work… sometimes they don't.

Affirmations tend to work much better if you believe them, while saying them. The first time I tried saying affirmations, I had a difficult time believing them as I said them. This is was something I wanted to believe, but felt I was lying to myself.
How was I supposed to change my life with affirmations when I didn't believe they were true?

Louise found that if you say affirmations with emotion, they work. If you say them with **a lot** of emotion, they work even better.

Louise also found that looking into the mirror while saying affirmations, was much more effective. There is something about looking yourself in the eye when you make a statement about yourself…It reaches down into your soul.

Repeating the affirmation also makes it more effective. After saying the affirmation several times, you may notice some emotion coming up. Keep looking yourself in the eye as you say it.. Let the emotion come. Let it go.
If tears come, keep repeating it.
Repeat it and keep looking yourself in the eye…until the tears stop.

POSITIVE AFFIRMATIONS HANDOUT

Once the tears stop....you will feel an inner peace. This is a form of self-therapy. This helps you reach down into your soul and release any and all emotional wounds that have been covered up for years. It may be anything from feeling unloved since childhood, or it may be an emotional issue you have with money.

If you don't feel any emotion after repeating the affirmation 10 times, don't worry. Just say it like you mean it. Maybe, there isn't a wound there to heal...
Or, maybe it's just not ready to be healed... today.

I have found that one affirmation will bring up no emotion one day ... and then bring a flood of tears another day. It all depends on you... Your consistency and where your soul is at in the healing process.

This technique is very easy...very effective...and very healing. It is also inexpensive.
It can help heal emotional wounds and set you free. All you need is a mirror, some affirmations, and your eyes...the window to your soul.

Attached are some printed affirmations. Review them and select the ones that you are drawn to. If you don't feel drawn to any...create your own.
If you like, you can use the following affirmations and re-word them... anything to help you feel comfortable saying them.

Say the affirmations 10 times a day, every day....(twice a day if you can) and see your life change...for the better.

Release your pain.
Release your anger.

Release your doubt.
Release your guilt.
See your emotional wounds be healed

Let the pain leave your heart…
Invite joy and inner peace to fill your heart.

See things come to you that you've always wanted.
You can have it…all.
You can have true love, joy, peace, health, success, wealth, and prosperity…

Total abundance…
You deserve it.
Try it. Pick a mirror, look yourself in the eye, and say, "I love you." You may feel silly at first, but if you're alone, who cares? It's about the healing and the peace you receive afterwards.

*Note: *Doing mirror work in a private, safe space is recommended.*
Affirmations from Louise Hay's book, *I Can Do It!*:
This is a new moment.
I am free to let go.
I move beyond my judgment. There is no right or wrong.
I forgive myself and others.
They did the best they could with the knowledge, understanding and awareness that they had at the time. I am strong to forgive and to let go. I let go of all fear.
I take loving care of my inner child.
I am safe and free.
I take responsibility of my own life.
I am willing to go beyond my own limitations.

My spiritual growth is lifting me to my highest good.

I am always willing to take the next step for my highest good.

I give myself permission to let go.

I am limitless.

I love and appreciate my body.

Money flows into my life in an abundant way.

I allow my body to return to its natural vibrant health.

I honor my body and take good care of it.

I radiate love, and love fills my life.

I am discovering and using my current and new talents.

Wonderful new doors are opening for me all the time.

I am in the process of positive, healthy change and I deserve the best

HEALTH – LOUISE HAY

I am grateful to be alive today!

I am constantly discovering new ways to improve my health and the health of others.

I give my body what it needs on every level.

I balance my life equally in work, rest and play.

I am willing to ask for help when I need it.

I trust my intuition. I listen to it and act on it now and always.

I help others.

I am grateful for my body. I love life!

My mind is full of pleasant thoughts.

FORGIVENESS – LOUISE HAY

I listen to my feelings. I am gentle with myself. My feelings are my friends and guide.

The past is over. The power is now.

I claim my own power.

I am free from the past. I move with joy into the now.

I get help when I need it from various sources. My support system is strong and loving.

I release old, negative beliefs and patterns. I let them go with ease.

I am open to new, positive beliefs and patterns. I accept them with ease.

I am forgiving, loving, gentle, and kind. I know that life loves me.

I forgive myself. I forgive others.

I am living the best way I know how.

I let others be who they are.

I love who I am.

It is safe for me to move into love.

I have and use my forgiveness, courage, gratitude, love, and humor.

I forgive everyone in my past for all perceived wrongs. I release them with love.

All of the changes that lie before me are positive ones. I am safe.

PROSPERITY – LOUSIE HAY

My income is constantly increasing.

I prosper wherever I turn.

I am open and receptive to all good and abundance in the universe. Thank you, life!

I am a magnet for money.

Prosperity of every kind is drawn to me.

I think big and allow myself to accept even more good from life.

Money comes to me in expected and unexpected ways.

I have unlimited choices. Opportunities are everywhere.

We are here to bless and prosper each other.

I now do work I love and I am well paid for it.

I appreciate the money that I have now and am open to receiving more.

I live in a loving, abundant, harmonious universe. I am grateful.

I am now willing to be open to the unlimited prosperity that exists everywhere.

I allow prosperity to enter my life on a higher level than ever before.

Life supplies all my needs in great abundance.

The law of attraction brings only good into my life.

I have prosperity thinking and my finances reflect this.

I delight in the financial security that is a constant in my life.

I am grateful for the good in my life.

Enormous wealth and abundance are available to me now. I am worthy and deserving of it.

I deserve the best and I accept the best now.

I allow money to flow joyously into my life.

My good comes from everywhere and everyone.

AFFIRMATIONS FOR CREATIVITY – LOUISE HAY

I release my creativity fully.

I am a creative being.

I have a creative mind.

I am creative in every area of my life.

My mind is creative.

I am the creator of my life.

Jillian's Personal Affirmations

I like short affirmations based on the phrase "I am." As I repeat these, I do my best to "become" what I'm affirming. Writing each affirmation ten times a day has changed my life!

I am Spirit.

I am purpose.

I am faith.

I am peace.

I am healthy.

I am lean.

I am nutrition.

I am inspiration.

I am money.

I am knowledge.

I am motivated.

I am promoted.

I am productive.

I am wealth.

I am creator.

I am trust.

I am truth.

I am joy.

I am fit.

I am strong.

I am wellness.

I am success.

I am healer.

I am inner authority.

I am healed.

I am whole.

I am respected.

I am prosperity.

I am healthy relationship.

I am value.

I am valued.

I am forgiveness.

I am forgiven.

I am inner power.

I am inner strength.

I am clarity.

I am protected

I am fun.

I am more than good enough.

I am connection.

I am love.

I am loved.

I am respect.

I am in demand.

I am validated.

I am acceptance.

I am accepted.

I am boundaries.

I am knowingness.

I am guided.

I am honor.

I am laughter.

I am deserving of all good.

I am receiving all good.

I am passion.

I am gratitude.

CHAKRA LIST handout

CHAKRA ENERGY VORTEXES

Chakra	Meaning
1st – Base/Root	physical body, grounding, survival
2nd – Sacral	sexuality, emotions, vitality
3rd – Solar Plexus	power, self-empowerment
4th – Heart	love, acceptance, balance, surrender
5th – Throat	communication, expression, vocation
6th – Brow (3rd eye)	vision, intuition
7th – Crown	God, spirituality, consciousness

FENG SHUI handout

Definition: Feng Shui (pronounced "fung schway") means "wind" and "water"—two things that are ever-changing—like our lives!

What is it?   Arranging or enhancing your outer world to enhance your inner world.

Origin: China, thousands of years ago

Types: Form school: Arrangement of objects to improve chi flow. Compass school: Based on homeowner's birth information and the compass points (north, south, east, and west)

Chi   Energy (life force)

3 THINGS TO KEEP IN MIND
    * Live with what you love
    * Put safety and comfort first
    * Simplify and organize

Questions to Ask Yourself about Items in Your Environment

Do I love it?

Do I use it?

Do I need it?

Does it give me a good feeling when I look at it or use it?

BAGUA (life categories)

      *Health and Family

      *Career

      *Fame and Reputation

      *Knowledge, Skills and Self-cultivation

      *Wealth and Prosperity

      *Children and Creativity

      *Love and Relationships

      *Helpful People and Travel

      *Center (unity)

Health and Family Bagua

Enhance this bagua when you would like to:

Improve your health

Improve your social life

Improve your relationships with family and relatives

Increase your honesty

Increase forgiveness

    Use:

Healthy plants (soft or rounded leaves)

Silk flowers or plants that look healthy

Pictures depicting *your* idea of good health

Pictures of gardens and landscapes

Floral prints and stripes (linens, wallpaper, upholstery)

Wood (tables, chairs, bowls, etc.)

The number 4

Pictures of friends, family

Blue and green items

Quotes about honesty and forgiveness

Career Bagua

Enhance this bagua when you would like to:

Find purpose in your life

Change job or career

Use:

Water features (fountains, aquariums, etc.)

Pictures (bodies of water, pools, streams, lakes, ocean)

Objects that symbolize your career or items with your company name

The number 6

Mirrors, crystals, or items made of glass

Black or dark-colored items

Quotes about success or career

Fame and Reputation Bagua

Enhance this bagua when you would like to:

Have a good reputation

Get more recognition

Use:

Items that demonstrate accomplishments (diplomas, awards, certificates, trophies)

Good lighting (sunlight or electrical)

Pictures of people or animals

Items that come from animals (feathers, leather, etc.)

The number 1

Pictures or statues of people you respect
Items in any shade of red
Quotes about integrity, fame, and reputation

Knowledge, Skills and Self-Cultivation Bagua
Enhance this bagua when you would like to:
Be a student of some sort
Increase self-growth
Have more wisdom
Use:
Information (books, CDs, etc.)
Pictures of mountains or quiet places
Pictures of accomplished people
Black or royal blue items
The number 7
Quotes about meditation

Wealth and Prosperity Bagua
Enhance this bagua when you would like to:
Have more money
Raise money for some particular reason
Appreciate the prosperity in your life
Use:
Water features (preferably moving water)
Wind chimes, flags, and banners
Valuable possessions (antiques, art, crystal, coin collections)
Pictures of things that you'd like to buy
Gold, green, and purple items (you may also use red and blue)
The number 8
Quotes about gratitude, wealth, or prosperity

Children and Creativity Bagua

Enhance this bagua when you would like to:

Be more creative or think more creatively

Develop your inner child

Have a better relationship with your child

Get pregnant

Have more joy in your life

Use:

Creative, playful, or colorful objects

Toys or stuffed animals

Pictures of children or artwork made by children

Rocks, stones, pebbles

Shapes that are circular, or metal items

The number 3

White, yellow, or pastel-colored items

Quotes about joy, children, or creativity

Love and Relationships Bagua

Enhance this bagua when you would like to:

Develop a romantic relationship

Improve an existing relationship

Develop a relationship with yourself

Use:

Items associated with love or romance

Paired items such as candles, flowers, books, pictures, etc.

Romantic love notes, lingerie, etc.

Pictures of yourself or you and your loved one

The number 2

Red, pink, or white items

Quotes about love and romance

Helpful People and Travel Bagua
Enhance this bagua when you would like to:
Have more helpful people in your life (customers, clients, mentors, babysitters, etc.)

Travel

Be more spiritual

Use:
Artwork or pictures of angels, goddesses, teachers, etc.

Spiritual objects (rosary, crystal, Bible, prayer book)

Pictures of people who have been helpful to you

Pictures or brochures of places you'd like to visit or live

The number 5

White, gray, or black items

Quotes about heavenly experiences

Center Area Bagua
Enhance this bagua when you would like to:
Experience more unity / health (this bagua pulls all the others together)

Use:
Yellow or earth-tone colors

The number 9

Jillian Lambert – Feng Shui Consultant 512-965-4252
www.realhealthreallife.net

BENEFITS OF
LAUGHTER handout

What would the world be like without laughter? Can you imagine people walking around with no smiles and no laughter? There is so much seriousness in the world. We could all take a few moments to lighten up and laugh. What a release laughter can be for body, mind, and spirit.

Laughter benefits us because it:

*Relaxes the body

*Boosts immune system

*Releases "feel-good" endorphins

*Increases circulation (blood flow)

*Decreases stress

*Decreases fear

*Decreases pain

*Decreases stress hormones

*Increases joy

*Improves sense of well being

*Creates bonds between people

*Improves relationships

*Makes us more socially attractive

*Feels good!

*Changes your perspective from negative to more positive

*Helps people "let go"

*Helps us express true feelings

*Improves quality of all relationships

*Helps fight disease

*Lowers blood pressure

*Is a good cardio workout (increases oxygen usage)

*Helps the healing process

*Helps distract

*Is free entertainment!

SUMMARY handout

WELLNESS LIFESTYLE GOALS WORKSHEET
Fill in whatever your goal is for each category.

Body Composition: Lean tissue vs. fat tissue

GOAL:

Flexibility: Complete range of motion. Stretch all major muscle groups after exercise. Hold each stretch for ten seconds or more. This allows the oxygen to get into the muscle. The oxygen helps to rebuild the muscle stronger and better.

Recommendation: five to twenty minutes once per day, hold each stretch for ten seconds or longer.

GOAL:

Cardiovascular: Running, walking, hiking, swimming, aerobics, kickboxing, cycling, rebounding, etc. Fat starts to burn after the fifteen- to twenty-minute mark of exercise. (Your body burns glycogen until then.) Twenty to sixty minutes, four or five times per week

GOAL:

Strength Training: Weight machines, free weights, stability ball, resistance bands, etc. These activities strengthen all of the major muscle groups. Two or three times per week every other day, or alternate muscle groups every other day. Muscles need forty-eight hours of rest after you work them.

GOAL:

Balance: Stability and coordination. Tools to improve balance are stability ball, Bosu, wobbleboard, and coreboard. Yoga also helps improve balance.

GOAL:

Soul Activities/Relaxation: Yoga, tai chi, meditation, reading, spirituality, art, massage, time in nature, bubble baths, hobbies, and so on.

GOAL:

Nutrition: Eat *lots* of raw fruits and vegetables. Eat healthy proteins, carbs, and fats.

Lean protein includes fish, tofu, chicken, and lean cuts of beef.

Healthy carbs: fruit, sprouted grain bread.

Healthy fats: avocados, coconut oil, flax seed oil, olive oil.

GOAL:

Water: Take your weight in pounds and divide in half. This is how many ounces you should drink daily. (For example, someone who weighs 120 lbs. should drink 60 ounces of water per day.)

GOAL:

Rest: Getting enough sleep keeps your fat burning process running efficiently. Lack of sleep slows the fat burning process. Get seven to nine hours of continuous sleep each night if possible.

GOAL:

Sunshine: The sun can help lift your mood, heal wounds, benefit some forms of acne eczema, and is also the best source of vitamin D. Get fifteen to twenty minutes of early morning sunshine each day.

GOAL:

Nature: Nature calms and heals us. Get out in nature at least once or twice a week—more often if possible. Time alone to think is very beneficial to your mental state and your physical well-being. This quiet time can be used to sort out problems, create new ideas, or just relax.

GOAL:

Positivity: A positive attitude makes a big difference in how you cope with life. Look on the bright side and see the good in things. Positive thinking is a great boost for your health. See positive. Think positive. Speak positive. Be positive.

CPSIA information can be obtained at www.ICGtesting.com
Printed in the USA
BVOW031326020412

286649BV00005B/24/P